Uplift

PRACTICAL AND REASSURING ADVICE FROM BREAST CANCER SURVIVORS

BARBARA DELINSKY

PIATKUS

Copyright © 2001 by Barbara Delinsky Charitable Foundation for Breast Cancer Research

First published in the UK in 2002 by
Judy Piatkus (Publishers) Limited
5 Windmill Street
London W1T 2JA
e-mail: info@piatkus.co.uk

First published in the USA in 2002 by Pocket Books, A division of Simon & Schuster, Inc.

The moral right of the author has been asserted

A catalogue record for this book is available from the British Library

ISBN 0 7499 2337 7

This book has been printed on paper manufactured with respect for the environment, using wood from managed sustainable resources

Data manipulation by Phoenix Photosetting, Chatham, Kent
Printed and bound in Great Britain by Mackays Ltd, Chatham, Kent

Contents

Foreword   v

1 **On Diagnosis:** First Things First   1

2 **Losing a Breast:** Practical and Emotional   17

3 **Radiotherapy:** Soaking Up the Rays   33

4 **Chemo and Hair:** Mane Matters   45

5 **Chemo and Everything Else:** A Smorgasbord   65

6 **Taking the Reins:** Regaining Control   77

7 **Family:** Our Inheritance   95

8 **Friends:** We Pick 'Em   111

9 **The Workplace:** Making It User-Friendly   125

10 **Support Groups:** From Traditional to Offbeat   139

11 **Humour:** You Have to Laugh . . .   153

12 **Men:** By, For and About   165

13 **Exercise:** Making the Body Better   185

14 **Religion:** Bringing in the Big Guns   195

15 **Pure Uplift:** Wrapping It Up with a Bow   203

Acknowledgements   219

An Invitation from *UPLIFT*   223

Foreword

I am no bra-burner. I'm far too private a person for that. I've always been content working behind the scenes for the causes in which I believe. As a writer I've had the luxury of letting my characters do my bidding, whether that meant advocating safe sex, or open-mindedness, or the beauty of small-town life. I've been known to switch hairdressers when one takes to gushing on *ad nauseam* about my books, and I refuse to shop in bookshops where the booksellers hover so that I can't browse like a normal everyday person. Because I *am* a normal everyday person. And I like my anonymity.

For that reason, UPLIFT is an aberration for me. But if ever a cause was near and dear to my heart – and therefore worth the risk of putting my private self out there – breast cancer is it.

Breast cancer has been a player in my life since 1950, give or take. I can't tell you for sure, because my mother's hospital records don't go back far enough. When my sisters and I petitioned for a copy of them several years ago, the earliest ones we received were from 1951. That year, we were aged eight, six (me) and five. According to what we've since learned from the occasional relative or friend, our mother was diagnosed two or three years before that.

We were ten, eight and seven when she died, but it wasn't until we were in our late teens that we learned she'd had breast cancer. It took my dad that long to say the word 'cancer', let alone 'breast'. Things were different back in the forties and fifties, and it wasn't just

v

my father. One of the early submitters to *UPLIFT*, Elinor Farber, who experienced breast cancer through her mother, had a similar experience.

"My mother was diagnosed with breast cancer 45 years ago. Since there were no mammograms at that time, she was diagnosed with the help of a 'fluoroscope' machine. She had a radical mastectomy, followed by a series of X-ray treatments. There was no radiotherapy available back then. I was 12 or 13 at the time. My sister, three years older than me, and I were both told of my mother's condition in hushed tones, and we were sworn to secrecy. I remember the panic and confusion that I felt. My mother, God bless her, lived for more than 30 years after her surgery, but she never spoke of her condition. She endured everything without the support of friends and neighbours, who were not told. I am so happy that breast cancer is no longer kept a dark secret. There is so much support now for women like my mother."

Indeed, there is. *UPLIFT* is a prime example of that. How did the book come to be? As a novelist firmly ensconced in fiction, I simply didn't think to write it – until the day last summer when I received one more note about Katherine Evans. Katherine is a character in one of my novels, *Coast Road*. She is the best friend of Rachel, the heroine, who is hurt in a car accident and lies in a coma through much of the book. Katherine is the one who notifies Rachel's ex-husband about the accident and who tells him what Rachel's life has been like in the years since they divorced. Katherine also happens to be a breast cancer survivor, though the reader doesn't learn this until halfway through the book, well after Katherine has been established as a woman who is vibrant and active, smart, attractive and successful. At that point, we realise that she is grappling with the sexual ramifications of having had a bilateral mastectomy.

Readers have been applauding Katherine in their letters to me since *Coast Road* was first published in the summer of 1998. When I received that note last summer, the idea hit, and, in an instant, *UPLIFT* was born. In that instant, I knew that I wanted to write a book about all the other Katherines out there, because my readers seemed so hungry for it. They liked Katherine being upbeat. They liked her having a productive life and not being solely defined by having had breast cancer. They liked her thriving physically. They said that she was an inspiration to them.

We are surrounded by people with a similar potential to inspire us. The problem is that we don't know it. We don't see all the women who have experienced breast cancer and moved on, whose lives are filled to overflowing with good stuff that has nothing to do with disease. When it comes to breast cancer, we hear about two kinds of women – those who are activists, often celebrities, and those who die.

Katherine is alive. I'm alive. Millions of other women are alive. If nothing else, this is what *UPLIFT* is about. Studies have shown that women consistently overestimate their risk of dying of breast cancer. No doubt, one of the reasons for this is that they've heard only about the Linda McCartneys of the world. They haven't heard about the Diane Cottings, the Ellie Anbinders, the Helen Kellys or the Asha Mevlanas. They haven't heard about the Billie Loops, the Carolyn Steins or the Willie Mae Ashleys. They haven't heard about the Barbara Delinskys.

I was diagnosed with breast cancer in 1994. Like so many women with a family history of the disease, I'd been waiting for it. Since I had been watched closely over the years, my cancer was caught early, picked up by a mammogram well before it was palpable. I had radiation the first year, then, when microscopic spots were found on the other breast the following year, a bilateral mastectomy and reconstruction. I told no one apart from my family and a handful of friends about any of this.

There were reasons why I was silent. None had to do with embarrassment. Anyone who has ever read my books knows that I have no trouble saying the word "breast". I certainly don't feel less of a person, or less of a woman, for having had breast cancer. Nor do I feel in any way responsible for bringing it on – though, years ago, this was indeed what women felt. No, I followed the "rules" and breastfed my babies, kept my weight down, took regular exercise and ate broccoli. I also knew that, in truth, nothing I did was going to change something that might well be embedded in my DNA.

I suppose I could say that I kept my secret out of fear that it would hurt my career, and there was a bit of truth in that. But it wasn't the main reason.

The main reason why I didn't tell anyone outside that close circle of family and friends was that I didn't want to be seen as ill. I'd had something bad removed from my body. It was gone. I was well. I was writing up a storm, as prolific as always, and this, more than anything, eased the emotional fallout of knowing that I'd had *IT*. When I went out, when I was with friends or colleagues, I didn't want their questions, however caring or wellmeaning. I didn't want expressions of sympathy – or worse, pity. They would have been inappropriate and would have only cast an unnecessary pall over my day. I was enjoying life too much to be talking cancer all the time.

Then why am I going public now? Perhaps because I'm far enough away from my diagnosis to know that others will know, as I do, that the cancer has gone. Perhaps because I'm established enough in my career to know that publishers will buy my books and readers will read them whether I have a cold, a canker or a cancer. Perhaps simply because I've become bolder since turning 50, so much bolder that I don't *care* who thinks what.

Actually, it's something else. In that "Eureka!" moment last summer, when *The Vineyard* was on the *New York Times* bestseller list and yet one more reader wrote to me about Katherine and *Coast Road*, I realised that I had the ears of millions of women and because of that *I could make a difference*. My readers look at my picture on book covers or talk with me at book signings, and, like Katherine, see a woman who is healthy, vibrant and strong. Telling them that I've had breast cancer and not only have recovered but am stronger than ever could make a difference to *them*. Additionally, there were three technical facts. First, I had the know-how to write a book. Second, I had the contacts to get it in print. Third, thanks to the success of my fiction, I could afford to donate all of my proceeds to breast cancer research.

In that pivotal moment, it struck me that helping women with breast cancer, and in doing so raising money for research, was what I wanted to do more than anything else.

From the start, I knew just what the book would be. It would be the support group that I had never joined but could have used, the one that offered all the practical little secrets to survival that have nothing to do with doctors, machines or drugs and everything to do with women helping women. But as support groups went, it would be unique in that it could be joined in total privacy, at any time of day or night, and selectively. It could also be consulted by the other people in our lives who are so important to us – our family, our friends, our colleagues. If they wanted to know how to help us – or how to help themselves through a rough period – this support group in book form would tell them.

I knew that I wanted my book to be written by women of every age and walk of life, because breast cancer doesn't discriminate. I wanted to give those women a voice, and I wanted to hear what they had to say myself — but only if it was positive. Time and again, I'd read studies showing the correlation between a positive attitude and the success of treatment. As far as I'm concerned, there is a correlation between a positive attitude and success in *life*. But still, when it came to breast cancer and the headlines in newspapers, the word was negative far more often than not. I'd read those headlines. We all have. Now I wanted to hear uplifting stories. I felt it was time to make the statement that . . . actually, Jane Vaughan, who was diagnosed in 1991 at the age of 53, said it best: "The morning I came round after the operation, I knew no one who had ever had breast cancer. I assumed that everyone who had it died. By mid-morning, friends who'd had breast cancer began coming out of the woodwork. I was amazed. And appalled that no one had told me that women actually could live."

So there it was. *UPLIFT* had a face. In hindsight, I had no idea how much work was involved in a project of this scope — not that it would have discouraged me if I had known. From the minute I conceived of this book, it was a passion for me. So I set to it, writing a detailed description of the project and a wide-ranging list of questions to spark the imagination of contributors. My assistant, Wendy Page, gave crucial help with this, as did my webmaster, Claire Marino, who took the material we'd written and designed a website that displayed it clearly and appealingly, with a submission form right there at the end.

One doesn't get submissions, though, without letting people know that a project exists. I began with a direct solicitation to my mailing list, which consists of the names of readers who have contacted me since my first book was published more than 20 years ago. My letter described *UPLIFT* and gave contact information — and the network began to grow. These readers told friends and relatives about the project. Some told reporters from their local papers, who wrote stories, which spread the word further. Others told their oncology nurses, who passed the information on to other survivors, who passed the information on to even more people. Friends and readers sent me the names of yet more contacts, which my assistant pursued. We sent out information on a daily basis.

UPLIFT doesn't pretend to be a scientific study. Once my initial mailing was complete, I could no more control who learned about the project than I could control who chose to respond. The guidelines made it clear that the book would contain positives, rather than negatives, so nay-sayers no doubt passed on it. Likewise, the heavy concentration of recently diagnosed women suggests that those still visiting cancer centres on a regular basis were more apt to see the *UPLIFT* material on display there than those whose cancer experience was far in the past.

Fellow writers were instrumental in spreading the word about *UP-LIFT* – from Elaine Raco Chase, who e-mailed her extensive mailing list, to Sandra Brown, who posted a note on her website, to Dorothea Benton Frank, who took time from a speech she was giving to distribute *UPLIFT* material at a lunch for breast cancer survivors. The latter was probably the closest brush that *UPLIFT* had with traditional breast cancer organisations. From the start, I wanted this to be a grass-roots effort. I wanted women like me, who are not typical activists, to have their say.

Submissions arrived in one of three ways: via the website, via e-mail or via the post. Some respondents followed the guidelines to the letter; others went off in a different direction. I was startled by the sheer length of some of the submissions – as long as *ten typed pages*, and that's not counting those who sent entire chapters from their diaries! Some of the material was funny, some practical, some simply and solely uplifting. Jeryl Abelmann, who was diagnosed in 1986 at the age of 46, put it well in the handwritten note that prefaced her very normal-length submission: "Longer than a word . . . shorter than a thesis . . . from the heart!"

Submissions began arriving in mid-October. By mid-December, patterns had emerged. Certain topics, like hair loss, were hot ones. But as a cancer survivor who had never had chemo, I wanted to know about other things, too. So I finetuned the guidelines to encourage a broader response. At the same time, I added questions on exercise and questions on the role of men in survivors' lives.

These questions yielded enthusiastic responses, particularly on the matter of men, which led to another modification. In January, with barely six weeks left in the submission process, I e-mailed all of those who had already submitted and invited the men in their lives to send along their own thoughts. As a result of the response to this e-mail, there is a specific chapter in *UPLIFT* by, for, and about men.

January became February. Just when I was thinking that I'd seen and read everything there was to be said on a topic, survivors would prove me wrong. Closing the submission phase at the end of February was hard to do, but it was necessary if I hoped to get the finished book to the publishers by the middle of May.

All told, I had more submissions than I'd ever hoped to receive. Though some were from friends and relatives of survivors, the bulk were from survivors themselves. They ranged in age at the time of diagnosis from 18 to 80, and some were diagnosed as long ago as 1954.

Reading the submissions took several weeks. I selected those that were consistent with the spirit of the book and typed them up – no mean feat, since some submissions contained upwards of a dozen separate elements. After printing out all the many pages, I literally cut the submissions up, so that I was left with strips of paper, each bearing a single entry and the name of its author.

Then the fun began. I put chapter signs around my dining-room table, like place settings for guests, and walked around and around, back and forth, putting those strips of paper into the appropriate piles. There was overlap; my chapters were far from mutually exclusive. A funny story about wigs, for instance (and there are *tons* of those), could easily work in a chapter on hair loss or one on humour. So I put some in the first and some in the second. It was the same with submissions on regaining control and on staying positive; some thoughts definitely bear repeating, albeit in different women's voices. As the sorting went on and certain piles grew too large for a single chapter, I divided those submissions up into smaller topics.

Initially, I had hoped to give clever little titles to each of the chapters. But working now with the actual submissions, I realised that it was more important that readers knew exactly what a chapter was about. Not every women needs chemo, or radiotherapy, or a mastectomy. If a woman is grappling with lumpectomy and radiotherapy, she doesn't need to hear about something she won't experience, like losing her hair. Push her too far when she's already fraught, and she could freak out.

I know this. I've been there. When I was first diagnosed, the treatment plan was for a re-excision and radiotherapy. Yet, in the midst of those seemingly endless hours waiting in examining rooms for the various doctors to appear, the nurse came in to explain the use of drainage tubes. I'd been pretty together up to that point, but I came close to losing it then. My husband, who was with me, will attest to the fact that I went deathly pale. *"No one told me about drainage tubes!"* I fairly yelled. The nurse said kindly, "But you will have to deal with them after you've had your operation." I cried, *"I'm only having a re-excision!"* She paused, then asked, "Only a re-excision?" When I nodded, she apologised, packed up her demo tubes, and left. Mind you, I did deal with drainage tubes after my operation the following year, and they weren't so bad. But I was ready for them then; I hadn't been ready the year before.

So UPLIFT is presented in a way that allows the reader to be selective. If a woman doesn't need chemo help, she doesn't have to read that chapter. If she isn't into religion, she can skip that one as well. If she doesn't have the peace of mind (a.k.a. attention span) to read for longer than five minutes at a time, UPLIFT allows for that, too.

This book is definitely informative, but its larger purpose is to be comforting. So it must be non-threatening. Beyond the clear labelling of chapters, this means the complete absence of medical talk. When I was going through treatment, I didn't read a single book, newspaper or magazine article on breast cancer. I was too busy *having* it. I was walking a fine line between panic and calm, and I simply couldn't risk reading something that would upset me.

Pat Baker, my friend and a breast cancer survivor since 1993, puts it well: "In almost every book on breast cancer, there are elements that frighten a patient. One becomes wary of picking up the material. But your effort can bring only comfort."

I'm trying, Pat, I'm trying. There are so many positive things to say, and so many women anxious to *say* them. Mind you, we aren't Pollyannas. We are definitely grounded in reality. Ask any one of us to discuss the pros and cons of various treatment options, and we'll give you an earful. But not here. No, definitely not here.

So, readers of UPLIFT can pick and choose – pick and choose what chapters they read, pick and choose what submissions within a chapter they read, even pick and choose what tips they want to follow. On certain topics, those cover the whole spectrum. For instance, some women swear that going to chemo on a full stomach works best, while others advise eating lightly beforehand. Some women swear that joining a support group was the best thing they ever did, while others say that they did just fine without.

If this is confusing to readers, I apologise. All bodies are different; some stomachs will settle with cream crackers, while others need a chocolate milkshake. Likewise, all *people* are different; some thrive on joining groups, while others have neither the time nor the desire to belong to one. The point is that there are choices. If one option doesn't work, another will. There are no rights and wrongs here. When readers are feeling overwhelmed, they need to know that *there is a solution*. The hundreds of women who've submitted to *UPLIFT* are proof of that.

Orchestrating *UPLIFT* has been an incredible experience for me. For starters, in picking a name for the project to coincide with a web address, I learned more about trademark law than I ever wanted to know. Then there were the submitters to *UPLIFT*, women and men whose names and experiences became as familiar to me as those of my neighbours and whose enthusiasm has been a highlight of this project for me. I would also be remiss if I didn't mention the days when I shamelessly touted the book to my publisher – shamelessly, because for the first time in my career, I could brazenly promote one of my books, since there was absolutely no money in it for me. I still get a rush from that.

In truth, though, putting *UPLIFT* together hasn't always been easy. I was never one to fill my day with cancer. During all those years waiting for it to hit, I did what I had to medically, then went on with the rest of my life. Suddenly, with *UPLIFT*, I was immersed in cancer as I never had been when I was being treated, and it was hard. I have to confess that there were days last autumn when I wondered whether I could do this – whether I could live and breathe the disease for the months that it would take to secure submissions and put together the book.

That fear passed, largely because of the wonderful people whose words constitute the body of this book. These people are upbeat. They are resourceful. They are intelligent, friendly and warm. They are generous. And they are funny. Mostly, though, I was time and again humbled by their eagerness to share their experiences and their hope of making things easier for others.

I close this foreword by quoting three such extraordinary women. Corinne Wood, who was diagnosed in 1997 at the age of 42, wrote, "Since I made my story public, not a week has passed without people coming to me seeking information or wanting to share their experience. The impassioned testimonials I hear from husbands, wives, sisters, daughters and friends help me to know I made the right decision in sharing my story. A generation ago, most people didn't talk about breast cancer. Many women suffered in silence, frustrated and alone, without access to information, advice or community support. We need to tell our stories. We need to humanise this disease. There is no shame in breast cancer; I want women to be proud to say, 'I am a breast cancer survivor. I beat this disease, and so can you!' "

Sheri Goodman, a social worker, who was diagnosed in 1999 at the age of 50, wrote, "Breast cancer is no longer a covert disease that is accompanied by embarrassment or shame. It is a disease that strikes regardless of age, race and socio-economic status, and we can no longer ignore its presence. It is through the stories of breast cancer survivors that we are so well informed on this issue. I am only one survivor, but I represent the many who have not yet spoken. I am sharing my story now to show that there is indeed life after breast cancer. I am a wife, a mother, a sister, an aunt, a friend, a social worker . . . and will someday be a grandmother. Yes, I am a survivor. We all are."

And finally, Sallie Burdine, a survivor and mother of three young children, wrote, "I've often played this little mental game with myself in a crowded place like a shopping centre or an airport. I imagine myself yelling out, 'Hey! Who here has breast cancer? Put your hands up!' And then maybe four or five women will slowly stop talking, walking or whatever and look at me and raise their hands. We will simply smile warmly at one another, as if to say, 'We're okay, we're not alone, we can do this.' And then everyone goes about their business, and I imagine we're all just a little bit stronger."

Here, then, is *UPLIFT*.

Barbara Delinsky
June 2001

1 · On Diagnosis

First Things First

Where was I when I learned that I had breast cancer? I will never forget it. I was exercising at home when my surgeon rang to say that the results of my biopsy were in and that the tiny little granules she had removed from my breast were malignant. *She told you that on the phone?* Indeed, she did. It was just the right thing for me, and she knew it. She and I had been through biopsies together before. She knew that my mother had had breast cancer and that I'd been expecting it. She knew that the best approach to take with me would be the understated one. She said, "The cure rate for this is 99.5 per cent. Here is what I recommend . . ."

I listened. Then I hung up the phone and called my husband. Then I finished my exercise routine. In doing that, I was showing myself that I was healthy and strong, cancer and all. I needed to minimise the impact of what I'd learned . . . because I knew that with a diagnosis of breast cancer, a part of my life had changed for ever.

I was shaky – and what frightened me most wasn't the prospect of having a re-excision and radiotherapy. It was phoning our three sons, who were in three different towns studying at college. I went about making dinner, a crucial same old routine, as I put through those calls, and as I talked to each son I had the first of many cancer experiences that weren't nearly as bad as I'd imagined. "Curable" was the word I stressed. My confidence was contagious.

Making Decisions

"When I was first diagnosed, I knew pretty much nothing about breast cancer – except that I didn't want it! By learning everything I could, I started to calm down, sort things out and actively make decisions. Knowledge is power. It definitely makes you feel a little bit more in control of your life."
Deborah Lambert; diagnosed in 2000 at the age of 47; medical secretary

"The first thing I did when the doctor told me I had breast cancer was to sit down, since I was weak in the knees, then to get a pen and paper. As a teacher I needed to get it all written down, to get it right. That served to calm me immediately."
Christine Foutris; diagnosed in 1999 at the age of 49; teacher

"When I came round after a lumpectomy and learned that I had breast cancer, I was in shock. To show how little I knew, when my husband was visiting and offered me a sip from his drink, I declined, saying that we didn't know if he could catch cancer from my germs. After he left, I picked up a book that a friend had left. Opening it at random, my eyes caught the words, 'A cancerous cell is, in fact, a weak and confused cell.' That made both of us, I thought, and laughed heartily."
Carol Pasternak; diagnosed in 1986 at the age of 47; artist

"I was devastated when I got the diagnosis of cancer. I'd had my mammogram faithfully every year. I went home to prepare dinner in a sort of shock. As I stood at the cooker I worried about what was going to happen and how I could handle it. Then, suddenly, a feeling of calm and peace came over me, and an inner voice said, 'You will be all right.' From that moment on, I knew I would survive."
Wendy Golab; diagnosed in 2000 at the age of 63; nurse

"Realise that a diagnosis of cancer does not mean instant doom. You have time to investigate, reflect, get several opinions and make careful decisions. Tell yourself this every morning, and tell everyone around you to keep telling it back to you."
Susan Stamberg; diagnosed in 1986 at the age of 48; journalist

"I didn't make any decisions about treatment until my children and significant other had been told. We all went to the surgeon's office together the next day. My children were all in their twenties. The district nurse and I gave one daughter a crash course so that she could change my dressings, and they all took turns driving me to my doctor's appointments and treatment. This reassured them that nothing was being kept from them."
Becky Honeycutt; diagnosed in 1995 at the age of 53; nurse

"One of the very first things I did, after the words 'cancer' and 'radiotherapy' were mentioned, was to get down to the local library to see what radiotherapy entailed."
Deb Haney; diagnosed in 1996 at the age of 48; administrative assistant, artist

"When I was first diagnosed, I wanted information immediately. I wanted to know which treatment plan was right for me. I rushed out and purchased the largest book on breast cancer I could find and read it twice. I sought the advice of trusted family, friends, doctors and breast cancer survivors. I made sure I was equipped with the best possible information, so that I could be my own best advocate."
Corinne Wood; diagnosed in 1997 at the age of 42; government official

"Treat your diagnosis as a business problem. Do research. Use the Internet and go through any literature available at the hospital. Feeling in control is pretty important, so begin with a notebook. The inside cover should have the name and telephone numbers of each of your carers (doctor, nurse, etc.) as they come on the scene. The notebook can be sectioned to keep track of doctor's appointments, definitions, outside advice, and so on."
Anne Jacobs; diagnosed in 1999 at the age of 62; managing partner, estate agency

"When I went to appointments after the diagnosis, I always had two or three of the children with me and sometimes all of them. They had so many questions to ask and also wanted to make sure I understood all the doctor was saying. After a while, I went with just my husband. When the doctor came in and saw only the two of us, he started hunting in all the cupboards and finally said, 'Okay,

where are they hiding?' We got a big chuckle out of that."
Sally Martel; diagnosed in 1996 at the age of 60; wife, mother, retired
accountant

"The hardest part of the whole mess was deciding what I wanted to
do. I struggled with the decision-making process. Finally a dear,
sweet lady said, 'Do your homework, make a decision, and don't
look back. You can deal with whatever is ahead of you when you get
to it.' She was right."
Mitzi Scarborough; diagnosed in 1999 at the age of 37; childminder

"How much do you really want to know? Be honest with yourself.
Once you have the answer and know what your learning style is,
find a survivor who is a match with you."
Kathy Weaver-Stark; diagnosed in 1991 at the age of 46; loss adjuster,
instructor

"I would have loved to talk to someone about all of this before I
had surgery and treatment. The worst part was my imagination. I
worried myself to death with chemotherapy horror stories. But it's
a lot like pregnancy; it's liveable, do-able."
Joy West; diagnosed in 2000 at the age of 34; advertising account co-
ordinator

"In deciding which option was best for me, I felt as though I was
looking at a Chinese menu. But what I found most comforting was
that no matter whom I talked to or what her own decision was,
each felt confident of her decision even years later. Women even
offered to show me their breasts. The idea of going to work without a bra began to sound pretty good."
Kathi Ward; diagnosed in 1994 at the age of 47; promotions executive

"During the diagnosis phase, go to a fertility clinic for advice if you
want to have children after treatment for breast cancer."
Alexandra Koffman; diagnosed in 1997 at the age of 40; nurse

"When you're first diagnosed, you may find yourself reading
books, watching videos, getting more and more information on
your options. The important thing to remember is that you need
to make the decision that's best for you. No one else can tell you

that what you have decided to do is wrong, because nothing is wrong, if it is what you want."
Glenda Chance; diagnosed in 2000 at the age of 38; housewife and mother

"Do what feels right for you. Don't let anyone talk you into anything."
Rhonda Sorrell; diagnosed in 1998 at the age of 43; special needs teacher

"Knowledge is power. The more educated you become, the less frightening the unknown is. Read, read and read more. It helps!"
Cathy Hanlon; diagnosed in 2000 at the age of 42; school researcher

"Twenty-one years ago, when I was diagnosed, many people recommended that I read a particular book on breast cancer. It happens that the author's husband had left her following her diagnosis. I remember thinking how depressing that was. My husband was there. He was worried about me, and I was worried about him, since he looked as though he'd been kicked in the stomach. I never had to even think about his leaving. I knew I was more to him than a pair of breasts, and any woman with a strong relationship should know so, too. It helped him that a family friend whose wife had recently had a mastectomy made the effort to talk to him. Marty isn't one who talks about his feelings much, but having a friend who'd been through it was good for him."
Lynne Rutenberg; diagnosed in 1980 at the age of 35; retired teacher

"Research everything about your disease. Ask questions. The ultimate decisions are yours to make. If you do your homework, you will feel that you have done the best for yourself and, ultimately, for all those who love and depend on you."
Christine Webber; diagnosed in 1998 at the age of 55; nurse

"Everyone handles traumatic situations differently. What is right for one can be wrong for another. I did everything I could not to dwell on my situation. I chose my doctors, got a second opinion, contacted a national cancer research body for the latest information, then I left it at that. A friend sent me a book with information

painstakingly highlighted for me -- I never read it. People sent me articles, which I never read. I dressed up for every appointment, so my doctors and nurses would see what I looked like when I was well and consider me a person who *would* be well. I was not in denial about having had breast cancer. Whenever I had a chance, I mentioned it to people. That was the promise I had made, the 'bargain' for my life . . . that I would spread the word that women had breast cancer and lived."
Jane Vaughan; diagnosed in 1991 at the age of 53; writer

"I strongly recommend joining a clinical trial. It is like having the undivided attention of a complete support team at all times."
Jacki Anthony; diagnosed in 1998 at the age of 48; nurse

"The four words that I live by: this too shall pass."
Suzanne Almond; diagnosed in 1996 at the age of 60; secretary

"Remember to thank your healthcare team as you navigate your way through the system of treatment. You would be surprised how much they worry about you as they plan your course of treatment."
Kathy Weaver-Stark; diagnosed in 1991 at the age of 46; loss adjuster, instructor

Helpful Little Tricks

"Take another person with you to your doctor's appointments. They can ask the questions you may forget to ask and can make sure things are explained properly. Also, take a list of questions with you, so you don't forget to ask the doctor something important. I know a woman who used to fax her questions in advance to her oncologist. Tape recorders are good for remembering the answers."
Sharon Irons Strempski; diagnosed in 1997 at the age of 52; nurse

"My mother and my husband were with me at every doctor's appointment after my diagnosis. My mum kept a spiral notebook with her at all times to take notes. When we went for the first consultation to discuss the results of the pathology report, my mother had written down all the words that could possibly describe a tumour. When the doctor began, Mum just started circling words. This helped all of us to concentrate on what the doctor was saying.

It was also helpful when reviewing it later and doing research."
Jennifer Wersal; diagnosed in 2000 at the age of 30; marketing executive

"After my diagnosis, my dear friend and neighbour Diane came to the rescue. Because my husband and I were numb and couldn't 'hear', Diane went with us to see three surgeons, a radiation oncologist and a reconstructive surgeon. She took notes and we discussed my options later. One surgeon also taped our consultation. I suggest to others that they take a tape recorder to all appointments, plus a 'Diane' – someone who loves you but can distance themselves."
Marianne Rennie; diagnosed in 1988 at the age of 39; cancer information specialist

"Take a little tape recorder with you when you have your initial consultations with the surgeon and oncologist. Even if you have a friend or family member with you, there is just too much information to remember. I was able to replay the tape for my mother and sister, and it helped to answer questions that I had later on. There is just too much emotion going on to have to rely on your memory for technical terms and procedures."
Deb Haney; diagnosed in 1996 at the age of 48; administrative assistant, artist

"When I was first diagnosed, a friend suggested I keep a diary of everything that was happening to me – what the doctor said, when and what the treatments were, and so on. I began doing that but found it to be too time-consuming. I was a pretty well-informed patient, and I didn't think I needed to concentrate on my cancer this way. Instead, I decided to keep a 'grateful diary'. Every day I wrote down five things that I was grateful for. Granted, some days it was difficult to meet that goal, but every day for nine months I wrote something. It was such a positive exercise during a difficult time in my life. When I read those entries now, they lift my spirits."
Susan Kowalski; diagnosed in 1997 at the age of 50; college executive staff assistant

"Form a 'phone tree'. Then you only have to give an update to one person. Otherwise, the phone rings off the hook!"
Stephanie King; friend of two survivors

Finding Early Support

"My husband was at home when I got the news. Our children were racing in the door from school and at the same time the radiologist on the phone was confirming to me that I had cancer. I hung up and felt swallowed up in confusion. My kids were rifling through the cupboards looking for snacks and my husband was looking at the terror on my face, knowing in his heart what had just been said on the phone without hearing a word. Our children were eight and ten, and we decided that they needed to know. I made appointments with their teachers and explained the circumstances. With four months left in the school year, I knew I would need their help and support. I felt as if I was assembling a team to go to war; it was empowering to have people on my side. When it came to the kids, we took them through each step separately so as not to overwhelm them – first surgery, then chemo, then radiation. Having the information gave them the power to talk about the experience as we all went through it."
Cindy Fiedler; diagnosed in 1988 at the age of 40; nurse, mother

"I never hid my diagnosis. I cannot stress enough the importance of being open. It is amazing how many people will be there for you. The support of others is one of the greatest healers around."
Dee Pobjoy; diagnosed in 1999 at the age of 41; sales clerk

"At the time of my diagnosis, there were several other women in town who'd had breast cancer. One of them was a good friend and tennis partner of mine. She called and gave me a lot of support and advice. This helped me tremendously."
Polly Briggs; diagnosed in 1987 at the age of 41; secretary

"On the day of my diagnosis, I phoned a friend who had gone through breast cancer three years before. She was very busy with work, but she gave me the time I needed. She told me that until I determined what my treatment should be, I would feel that I was totally out of control, but that once the decision had been made, it would feel as though a ton of bricks had been lifted from my shoulders. She was correct. I will always remember her last words. I said that I appreciated her time and long pep talk, and she said, 'You

know, this is therapy for me, too.' "
Caroline C. Hudnall; diagnosed in 1992 at the age of 55; retired court offical

"My surgeon told me I had breast cancer at 5 p.m. on a Monday and gave me until noon the next day to decide between mastectomy and lumpectomy. I knew what a mastectomy was, but I knew nothing about a lumpectomy. Frantic, I called two of my friends, each of whom had a friend who'd had breast cancer. Both of these women called me that night. They offered no opinions but did give me the knowledge I needed to make the right decision. They were absolutely wonderful with their support before, during, *and* after the surgery. They also helped me understand the process of radiotherapy. This is a scary experience, Without their help, it would have been much more stressful."
Rose Marie Clark; diagnosed in 1996 at the age of 50; retired

"When I was first diagnosed, I e-mailed a few friends to let them know. One friend who was not on my initial list e-mailed me to say, 'We're your friends in the bad times as well as the good!' After that, I gave my two closest friends permission to pass on my e-mail to anyone they felt it would help. The list grew over the next six months from 14 to over 200. Discovering that people truly care about me was wonderful."
Deb Haggerty; diagnosed in 1999 at the age of 51; professional speaker

"My feeling when I learned my diagnosis was, 'Why me? I have been a good person and had such a nasty marriage and things are finally good in my world. Why now?' I was scared and cried in the car park. My boyfriend, Jerry, held me tightly and kept reassuring me that my cancer was curable. After surgery, the cards and phone calls were not to be believed. My bosses sent flowers and two huge live lobsters, which I loved!"
Sharon Daniels; diagnosed in 2000 at the age of 49; hairdresser, wig shop owner

"Sleep didn't come easy to me after my diagnosis. Instead of sleeping pills, my husband and I started having a glass of wine before bedtime to help me relax. Every night while we drank wine, we talked, we read to each other and we played games. This became a special time together when we shared our feelings, fears and hopes

for the future."
Julie Crandall; diagnosed in 1998 at the age of 31; housewife and mother

"We got two kittens a few weeks before I learned I had cancer. They were confined to the spare bedroom. Whenever I was feeling down, I would go in and lie on the bed with them. They would climb all over me, cheering me up. My husband referred to my going in there as 'opening a can of kittens'."
Jeanne Sturdevant; diagnosed in 1990 at the age of 45; artist

"Being a mother, wife and nurse, I'd always been in the position of caring for everyone but myself. So I made an appointment with the social worker who was affiliated to the breast centre I went to. Now, I must confess, I'm not one to share my feelings with a perfect stranger, but somehow I felt this was the healthiest thing to do. Though it was awkward and uncomfortable at first, I visited this social worker regularly. This helped me keep things in perspective. As time passed, I looked forward to our visits as a time when I could speak of what I feared or celebrate my accomplishments."
Cindy Fiedler; diagnosed in 1998 at the age of 40; nurse, mother

Growing Bold

"When I came round in hospital after my mastectomy, the operating-room nurse was sitting by my bed. A breast cancer survivor herself, she had been sent by my surgeon. Her advice was, 'When you need something from someone, ask.' My generation of women was taught to 'suffer silently', not to complain or impose. An hour or so later, my husband rang up from his office to see how I was. I told him that I needed him, and he came immediately. Before the nurse's advice, I would have told my husband that I was okay – and then been miserable. Her advice has improved everything in my life!"
Jane Vaughan; diagnosed in 1991 at the age of 53; writer

"Write all your questions down before your doctor's appointment. Make sure your doctor listens to you and doesn't talk down to you. If necessary, change doctors until you get the right one."
Ellen Beth Simon; diagnosed in 1998 at the age of 41; lawyer

"If you think that something isn't right or hasn't been answered or resolved to your satisfaction, keep at it until you *are* satisfied – *every* step of the way! When I had doubts about the way a radiotherapist was setting me up for treatment, I asked for him not to work with me in the future. My request was respected. That was important."
Anne Jacobs; diagnosed in 1999 at the age of 62; managing partner, estate agency

"The mammography technician who helped prepare me for biopsy surgery was so kind that I have requested she do my mammograms each time I have gone back for follow-ups. As a result, she and I have become friends."
Jeanne Sturdevant; diagnosed in 1990 at the age of 45; artist

"If a needle wire localisation is being done before a biopsy or lumpectomy, ask if it can be done in the supine position. Most modern cancer centres can do this. I had to sit up for the first round, only minutes before my lumpectomy. With the discomfort of the procedure and anticipating the surgery afterwards, I passed out cold! My surgery was cancelled and I had to return for it a week later. The second time went much better. It was easier being able to lie down."
Donna Barnett; diagnosed in 1999 at the age of 40; nurse

"I refused to go back to the first oncologist I saw, because he made me feel like a piece of meat. The second one was very sensitive to my feelings. He made a note on my records that no male radiotherapists were to take care of me, and the female ones made a point of being busy with other things while I was undressing, thus making me feel less exposed. You have to speak up for yourself and let people know what your comfort levels are."
Sharon Irons Strempski; diagnosed in 1997 at the age of 52; nurse

"Get a second opinion if you are unhappy with the first one. Do some reading and speak up for what you want."
Mary Raffol; diagnosed in 1998 at the age of 44; teacher

"At no other time in your life will you have so much power and control over your own destiny; choose your health team well."
Kathy Weaver-Stark; diagnosed in 1991 at the age of 46; loss adjuster, instructor

"I became bold enough to leave my first surgeon and oncologist, because I didn't feel comfortable putting my life in their hands. At least, I still had *some* power."
Kathi Ward; diagnosed in 1994 at the age of 47; promotions executive

"My first oncologist asked whether I wanted to have treatment, since there was no guarantee that it would help. My husband and I left that doctor and found another, who said, 'You have a one in eleven chance, and you might as well be that one.' His positive attitude lifted our spirits. A year later, when my treatment was over and he told us there was no sign of cancer, I thanked him for saving my life. His reply was that my positive attitude had made the difference. 'You knew you were going to get better, and you did,' he said. Attitude is so important on everyone's part."
Florence Chandler; diagnosed in 1995 at the age of 66; retired hotelier

Attitude Indeed . . .

"The most constructive thing I did when I received my diagnosis was to continue to write out the invitations to my daughter's wedding."
Frances Gallello; diagnosed in 2000 at the age of 51; mental health assistant

"The best thing I did after being diagnosed was *not* to cancel a planned bicycle trip. It did more for my optimism than anything else could have done. Same thing with attending a neighbourhood party on the day I came home from hospital. I refused to hole up in self-pity."
Judith Ormond; diagnosed in 1996 at the age of 49; symphony musician – piccolo

"My husband, who is my best friend, took me for a walk in the woods the day I was told I had a malignancy in my breast. He knew that was where my spirit was most at peace."
Robin Smith; diagnosed in 2000 at the age of 53; microbiologist

"I cried a lot during the two weeks between learning I had breast cancer and having the operation. Once all the decisions were made and the operation over, though, I considered myself 'on the road to recovery' and I was determined not to cry or feel sorry for

myself. I've always been an optimistic person and was determined
to continue that way. I considered what was happening to my body
to be a temporary condition."
Patti R. Martinez; diagnosed in 1999 at the age of 54; estate agent

"Seven years ago, when I got my cancer diagnosis, I fell apart. I had
no one to tell, my children were away at college and I was by myself
in the country. I remember going straight to the barn to see my
animals. My main concern was who was going to take care of them
if I could not? My animals were the reason I was living in the country. They were part of my family. I went to visit a neighbour who was
93 years old at the time and I had every intention of telling her
what was wrong. When I walked into her house, though, she spoke
before I did. 'You know,' she said, 'some days God gives us a heavy
load to carry and we must do the best we can.' My neighbour died
the following Sunday, and I still remember what she said. This is
my eighth year since the diagnosis. My life has changed and I have
met wonderful people whom I would not have otherwise known."
Antonia Rhodes; diagnosed in 1993 at the age of 50; breast cancer
charity worker

"When I was diagnosed, I had just retired and we had many plans.
I found that continuing to work on those plans helped me to
realise that this was just a bump in the road."
Monetta Lockey; diagnosed in 1997 at the age of 59; retired teacher

"Even after my diagnosis, I went on a Caribbean cruise as planned.
I continued with my regular schedule as soon as possible, seeing as
many friends and relatives as possible so that they would know I
was alive and well."
Carol Hattler; diagnosed in 1999 at the age of 65; retired nurse

"When I was diagnosed with breast cancer, I took six months' leave of
absence from my job. During this time, amid surgery, chemotherapy
and radiotherapy, I discovered my creative side. I began to write
poetry."
Mary Platt; diagnosed in 1998 at the age of 47; radiology supervisor

"One strange thing – I cried when I was first diagnosed and never
cried after that. Now, I cry at so many things. I feel that it's healthy

to do so. But I don't cry for myself. Not ever."
Sheila Roper; diagnosed in 1995 at the age of 57; housewife

"When my doctor told me that I had breast cancer, I had a good cry. Then I decided that I wanted to live and would do everything necessary to achieve that goal."
Sandy Mark; diagnosed in 1998 at the age of 55; administrative assistant

"When I was diagnosed, I kept three bits of advice in mind. First, stay in control. Second, be informed. Third, keep a positive outlook. After my surgeries, chemotherapy and radiotherapy, I add a fourth to the list: be proud to be a survivor."
Helen Ann Kelly; diagnosed in 1996 at the age of 43; teacher

"My husband says that he got most of his comfort from me, because he felt that I was in control both of my disease and of the day-to-day workings of our lives. That was my goal – to keep everything at home operating as usual. The most contructive thing I did after hearing my diagnosis was to personally tell every friend, relative, neighbour and colleague of my diagnosis. As time passed, I kept everyone up to date with all the details, so that there would be no mystery or misunderstanding."
Deborah J. P. Schur; diagnosed in 1994 at the age of 43; sales rep

"A breast cancer diagnosis can be terrifying, especially because there is a lot of waiting – waiting for the mammogram results, waiting for the biopsy results, waiting to talk to the surgeon and plastic surgeon, and then waiting for the surgery. All this waiting can lead to a lot of stress and anxiety! It didn't take me long to realise that I had to take control or I would lose control. I believe the single most powerful thing I did to get through my breast cancer diagnosis was to concentrate on truly living and enjoying every day. For me this meant simply keeping very busy, doing things I enjoyed doing. The last thing I needed was time on my own. I took every opportunity I could to simply be with people – anybody and everybody. By forcing myself to be out in the world, surrounded by other people, I was forcing myself to look beyond myself. And did I keep busy! My husband and I took long bike rides, we went shopping, we went out for meals, we went away every weekend – to the beach, to the mountains, anywhere, while we waited. It sounds so simple, but by keeping busy and active, I was reminding myself that life does go on. I did not feel ill; I felt healthy and alive. It was liberating to feel in control of my actions and my mind."

Julie Crandall; diagnosed in 1998 at the age of 31; housewife and mother

"Being diagnosed at 24, married and taking care of a two year old can be overwhelming for anyone. Not me! When I found out I had cancer, I did not think I was going to die. I was just going to face the facts and beat this, and I did."

Candice Jaeger; diagnosed in 2000 at the age of 24; wife and mother

"I have always tried to live and eat healthily. Still, I found a lump in my breast. I had a mastectomy and reconstructive surgery. Since I am the mother of two daughters and have two grand-daughters, I participated in a clinical study. I thought that if my participation could help at least one other person, it would all be worth while."

Nancy Ellis; diagnosed in 2000 at the age of 53; quality control technician

"One year ago I was diagnosed
My life turned upside down
How do I feel about that?
I don't know.
Happy to be alive
I would be dead
If not for the check-up
How do I feel about that?
Grateful."

Cheryl Wilkinson; diagnosed in 1999 at the age of 45; fast-food worker

"From the beginning, set your mind on one thought: I will beat this. It will not beat me."

Susan Schultz; diagnosed in 1990 at the age of 41; special needs assistant

"What worked for me? Never ever, *ever* thinking I would not survive."

Eleanor Anbinder; diagnosed in 1991 at the age of 50; sales manager

2 · Losing a Breast

Practical and Emotional

What to do? Lumpectomy? Mastectomy? Single? Double? Reconstruction with saline implants? TRAM-flap reconstruction? *No* reconstruction?

So many questions, so many decisions. *UPLIFT* won't give you the answers. Nor does it discuss the medical merits of one procedure or another. It simply tells you of the decisions that different women made and why they are pleased with those choices.

I'm pleased with the choices I made. They were the right ones for me. As crass as it may sound, losing a breast was never something I spent much time thinking about. Before I was diagnosed, it was too *painful* a thought to dwell on. I had my mammograms and my physical examinations, did everything I could medically to ensure early detection. Then I blotted it out. I figured I'd deal with it when and if I had to.

When I was first diagnosed and my surgeon recommended a re-excision and radiotherapy, I happily went along with it. For those of you unfamiliar with the term, re-excision is a lumpectomy involving cells too small to be called a lump. My doctor predicted a high cure rate with this plan, and I had total faith in her. The following year, when cancerous cells were found in the other breast, she recommended mastectomy. Given that both of my breasts had now proved to be cancer-prone, I was content to get rid of them.

My husband was more torn. Not long ago, when I asked him about this, he confessed that the idea of mastectomy had initially frightened him. I'd sensed that at the time, based on his repeated urgings that I shouldn't rush into a decision. But he hadn't been living with the spectre of cancer all the years that I had. Once he realised how much it meant to me to deal with it once and for all, he never looked back. He has been totally supportive and has never shied away from looking at my new breasts. If he finds them any less attractive than the old ones, he's never let on. And let's be honest, girls – some things men simply can't hide.

No, I don't regret my decision to have the mastectomy. My only regret is that I didn't have it done the first year. This would have saved me the six weeks of radiotherapy then, not to mention the struggle with reconstruction that came from trying to stretch my irradiated tissue a year later. But we're all brilliant with hindsight. The truth is that I wasn't ready for a mastectomy that first year. If I'd done it then, I would have always wondered if it had been necessary. The bottom line here? I did what was right for me at the time.

That is what you all have to do. What was right for me isn't necessarily right for you. If you've just had a single mastectomy, you may want to skip the section on doubles. You've already made your decision; the surgery is over; second-guessing it won't accomplish anything except make you a nervous Nellie.

UPLIFT looks at the positive side of losing a breast, but make no mistake – surgery isn't fun. No one *wants* to have a mastectomy. No matter how you look at it, the procedure is barbaric. And I do miss my breasts. I miss the look of them, particularly in summer when women wear tank tops that show the gentlest curve of a breast. I miss them at night. They were sexual beings.

That said, I wouldn't want them back. They were lumpy. They were sore. They caused me worry for a long, long time. Then came cancer. I'd say that losing my breasts is a small price to pay for another 40 years of life. Of course, I may rethink that in 30 years when my joints are stiff, my back is bent and my daily worries centre around constipation . . .

The Dirty Deed

"Amazon women used to remove a breast in order to shoot their

arrows with better accuracy. I had breastfed all three of my sons and at 47 didn't need to have breasts any more."
Jane Royal-Davidson; diagnosed in 1996 at the age of 47; teacher

"My surgery was to be on 7th November – my birthday and my son David's birthday. I was turning 46, and he was turning 18. I said to him, 'I am so sorry that my operation is on our birthday.' His response was, 'Mum, I'm glad your surgery is going to be on our birthday. This is not a leg, or an arm or an eye. It is a breast. And, Mum, think of this as a rebirth. Because it *is* our birthday.' "
Jeryl Abelmann; diagnosed in 1986 at the age of 46; primary school teacher

"When my husband hugged me, I told him I was frightened. I shed a few tears. The image of how my breast would look after the surgery hit me. Charles reassured me that he would love me regardless of how it looked. When I apologised for crying, he said he was glad to see me finally acting in a 'normal' manner."
Sandy Williams; diagnosed in 1999 at the age of 51; children's public librarian

"As I prepared for my surgery I drew images of one-breasted women. Now why do they all tend to be warriors? I am a Sagittarian, and a mythical figure that has always held high significance for me is Chiron the centaur, the wounded healer. The version I created was Christon, a one-breasted female centaur, drawing back her bow unimpeded across the flattened right side of her chest. Yes, I've probably finally lost it, but paradoxically, along with the fear and sheer disbelief that I am actually about to have a breast cut off, I am feeling freer and more truly myself than I have for a long time!"
Christine McNamara; diagnosed in 2000 at the age of 54; retired director

"The morning after my surgery, I was determined to be normal, even though I could barely lift my arm. I put make-up on – the doctors were not going to see a sick woman when they came into my room. I think the surgeon and oncologist were very surprised!"
Marianne Rennie; diagnosed in 1988 at the age of 39; cancer information specialist

"There was a cleaners' strike at the hospital and my bathroom was filthy. So right after my operation I cleaned the bathroom with my right arm, holding the IV pole!"
Aileen Pandapas; diagnosed in 1989 at the age of 41; mother, volunteer, former secretary

"The day after my mastectomy, I was taken to the rehab room to begin reactivating the muscles affected by the surgery under my arm for the lymph node tests. During the wheelchair ride down several floors, I drooped and felt sorry for myself – an amputee without the strength to walk down the corridor by herself. Did I get yanked back to reality fast! An 18-year-old boy learning to walk with a wooden leg was supporting himself on the bars and falling again and again. An older man was learning to walk with two wooden legs while his anguished wife watched his stumbling attempts. A multiple sclerosis victim was trying to activate dying muscles. It hurt a little as I walked my fingers up the wall, but at least I didn't need to learn how to navigate without a vital appendage. After all, I had breastfed my three children. These breasts had fulfilled their purpose."
Lorraine J. Pakkala-Lintala; diagnosed in 1992 at the age of 62; editor, author

Clothes, Pillows and Bras . . .

"The daughter of a breast cancer survivor gave me a nightdress with buttons down the front to wear in the hospital. The morning after my operation, I had a wash and put on this bright nightdress. I felt feminine again. The button opening allowed me to deal with the drainage tubes."
Sheila Levine; diagnosed in 1992 at the age of 43; teacher

"My favourite piece of clothing right after surgery was my husband's T-shirt. It was so comfortable."
Barbara C. Sumner; diagnosed in 1982 at the age of 59; housewife

"I had a bilateral mastectomy and felt as though I was a tangle of tubing. I found that the easiest way to deal with the drainage tubes was to string all of them on a long shoelace and tie it around my waist."
Linda Dyer; diagnosed in 1993 at the age of 40; magazine editor

"I bought some large men's shirts to wear after my surgery. They were comfortable and easy to get in and out of."
Val Long; diagnosed in 1999 at the age of 47; administrative assistant

"Because I had mobility problems with my arm, I was too anxious to succeed in putting on a T-shirt. Well, I finally did it . . . but then I couldn't get it off! I live alone. I ended up wearing the T-shirt for a few days."
Judith Ormond; diagnosed in 1996 at the age of 49; symphony musician – piccolo

"What really helped after surgery was a foam wedge. I had a double mastectomy, reconstruction and hysterectomy all in one operation. So it wasn't easy to lie flat in bed. The foam wedge can be turned several ways to allow for easier positioning and more comfortable sleeping. I had also purchased three house dresses that had poppers up the front, top to bottom. They were easy to get in and out of, and were washable."
Gwen Loverink; diagnosed in 1994 at the age of 34; police dispatcher

"My mother made me a small pillow to put between my arm and ribcage for the days following my surgery. It made sleeping more comfortable. I was warmed by this loving gift, and have passed it, and other pillows, along to friends facing breast surgery."
Marcia Gibbons; diagnosed in 1991 at the age of 52; artist

"I had massages before surgery and resumed as soon after as I could. There are massage therapists trained to work with cancer patients."
Anne Jacobs; diagnosed in 1999 at the age of 62; managing partner, estate agency

"I applied a form of aloe vera gel to the incision every day. There were no puckers, red marks or problems at all."
Lorraine J. Pakkala-Lintala; diagnosed in 1992 at the age of 62; editor, author

"I didn't undress in front of anyone, and even with my husband it took me six months. He was fine with it, but I wasn't. It's good for

new patients to know that the scar fades and diminishes an awful lot."
Irene Louise; diagnosed in 1995 at the age of 41; retired PA

"My husband rigged up 'training equipment' for me. It was a clothesline and pulley over a clothes rod, so I could pull my arm up and exercise the arm muscles. It was in a walk-in wardrobe. That wardrobe became my sanctuary – a good place to hide, cry and swear."
Earlene Smith; diagnosed in 1985 at the age of 52; part-time postal worker

"After eight weeks post-op of not being able to raise my arms much, I went to physiotherapy. I have four children and I needed to be able to do things. Over the next month, I regained 98 per cent of my pre-surgery movement. However, when I got the green flag to drive, I was intimidated. I found that using a flat, square pillow between my body and the seat belt gave me a real security boost. I got a lot of funny looks from other drivers, but it was worth the independence I gained."
Linda Caradec; diagnosed in 1999 at the age of 41; microbiologist

"When my daughter arrived to take me home after my mastectomy, I made a bizarre joke about my double-breasted coat being useless now. She took in the situation in an instant. 'Welcome to reality,' she said. 'Shelly [her sister] and I have had to stuff our bras since we were 12.' Whipping the curtain around us, she yanked tissues from the box and started stuffing my empty bra cup. In no time she had constructed a size 38B. I was in awe of her expertise. 'I've had lots of practice,' she said smugly, and we went home."
Lorraine J. Pakkala-Lintala; diagnosed in 1992 at the age of 62; editor, author

"When I had my operation 20 years ago, I remember being afraid to look at my incision. Also, I wore a bra stuffed with Kleenex for *months* until the school nurse told me about a special shop where I could be fitted for a prosthesis. If she hadn't suggested it, I'd probably still be using Kleenex!"
Hope Cruickshank; diagnosed in 1975 at the age of 54; retired secretary

"The best purchase I made after my mastectomy was a good breast prosthesis. When I received my new breast form and walked out of the shop, I felt complete. My daughter said that I'd been going around with my head down and would not look at people. Wearing the new breast form, I held my head high. I knew that I looked like everyone else and I felt in balance again. No one had told me that I would feel *out* of balance after having one breast removed, but I did. I didn't realise how much until I got my prosthesis and the problem was solved."
A survivor; diagnosed in 2000 at the age of 50; teacher's assistant

"Being fitted for a prosthesis was quite interesting. The fitter explained that there are over five shapes of breasts. She found my shape, size and a corset-looking bra, and made me put it on then and there. The fit was perfect, a perfect three-pound balance. When I got dressed and left the fitting room, my daughters couldn't tell which was the new breast. We went out to a very fancy restaurant to celebrate."
Lorraine J. Pakkala-Lintala; diagnosed in 1992 at the age of 62; editor, author

"I refused to let the surgery get in my way. So six days after I got home, my friend and I went out to buy some pretty nightdresses. Though I couldn't stand up straight, the fresh air felt wonderful and I proved to myself that I could do it. Seven weeks after the surgery, I played golf. Hey, I could do that, too, and my right arm worked!"
E. Mary Lou Clauss; diagnosed in 1991 at the age of 55; housewife, retired nurse

"During my rehab, I thought I would never be able to use my left arm again. Well, let me tell you, that left arm is now used for carrying around five grandchildren and for swinging a golf club."
Joanne Bellontine; diagnosed in 1982 at the age of 39; recruitment consultant

"For five years following my mastectomy (without reconstruction), I had some pain or discomfort with my bras. Several months ago, the pain specialist at my GP's surgery suggested I try a sports bra. The place where I purchased my mastectomy bra did not have a sports bra on offer. So I went to the high street and purchased one there. At first, I pinned the prosthesis to the bra, since there was no pocket for it. Then one day I forgot to pin it in, and I was surprised at the end of the day to find that it had stayed in place all day with no problem. I love sports bras – I no longer have any pain or discomfort, the strap is out of the trench on my shoulder and they are not expensive."

Margaret Leggett; diagnosed in 1995 at the age of 58; retired personnel executive

"In 1985, I had a mastectomy. As I began to heal I knew it was time to buy a prosthesis, but I kept procrastinating, pretending I was too busy with the approaching holiday season. I found a comfortable blouse with a right-hand pocket where I could stuff Kleenex, so I bought half a dozen in various colours. I wore them to work with loose jackets to camouflage my lopsided figure. My husband, Ted, had been especially supportive throughout the preceding months, combining loving tenderness with pragmatism, but I felt his attention was waning. One Saturday he said, 'Come on, we're going shopping. No questions or excuses!' He escorted me into an exclusive lingerie shop. Stylish women were trying on sheer negligees and lacy underwear. I felt like a fish in a bicycle shop. Then Ted asked for someone by name and I realised he had arranged for an appointment. A lady showed me into a private changing room and fitted me for my prosthesis and mastectomy bras. She couldn't have been kinder or more professional. I joined Ted at the cash register as she brought my purchases – in a plain white box – from the back room. 'Gift wrap them, please,' Ted said, getting out his credit card. In front of the whole shop, he handed me the gaily wrapped package, gave me a deep kiss and winked. 'Merry Christmas!' Now, even after years of enjoying my reconstructed bustline, I still remember these cherished gifts."

Nancy Sena; diagnosed in 1985 at the age of 46; retired counsellor

All in the Family

"My 15-year-old daughter's response to my approaching mastectomy? 'So you'll be uni-boobed!' "

Mindy Greenside; diagnosed in 2000 at the age of 48; midwife

"My husband emptied and measured the drainage tubes when I got home from the hospital. He was there for me all the time."
Rebecca Clarkson; diagnosed in 1997 at the age of 45; road transport worker

"My grandmother was an amazing lady. At the age of 89, she had a double mastectomy. Less than two hours after the surgery, she was out of the recovery room and being wheeled into her room. She immediately began giving orders. 'My teeth are in that drawer – I need them.' 'Where is the telephone – I want to call my friend Jenny to tell her that the food at this hospital is better than the food at her hospital.' She recovered quickly and came home several days later. I went with her to be fitted for her prostheses. She had always been a very large-breasted woman and she now chose a smaller size. Once the prostheses arrived in the post, she wore them all the time. She said that if she had known they would look so much better, she would have done this years ago!"
Marianne McCaskill; granddaughter of Anita Lundberg

"I quickly lost my self-consciousness about undressing in front of others, because my husband and my neighbour changed my bandages. They stood there gazing and talking about how good it looked, and this was good for me, because I hadn't been afraid of the word 'cancer', but of how my husband would accept my disfigurement. I should have known better, as he loved me, not only my breast. He was my rock. He never let me think about losing a breast, just about beating the odds."
Jacqueline Durant; diagnosed in 1994 at the age of 68; retired

"My husband was wonderful. His sense of humour helped me tremendously. He frequently hid my prosthesis or walked around with it on his prematurely balding head. He made it comfortable for all six of the children to look at the prosthesis, feel it and look at me without it. He was so wonderful with my body that I never felt less of a woman. We were both so grateful that I was alive that losing a breast was not devastating."
Cornelia Doherty; diagnosed in 1985 at the age of 45; mother, widow, speaker

"To all women who are single or divorced and have had breast cancer, do not be afraid. You are not just a breast. You are a beautiful woman and will find a loving man who will love you for you. Real men don't care about your scars. Everyone has baggage."

Miriam Cooper; diagnosed in 1982 at the age of 36; mother, volunteer, estate agent

"Day after day following my mastectomy, I looked in the mirror and saw this disfigured woman, and I became depressed. My husband, noting the change in me, asked what was wrong. When I told him how I felt about myself, he took me in his arms and said, 'I didn't marry you 30 years ago because you had two breasts. I married you because I loved you, and I will love you till the day I die, whether you have one breast or none.' This was what I needed to hear to become a whole person once again."

Frances Meadow; diagnosed in 1973 at the age of 50; retired business owner

"Neither my husband nor I misses my breasts. We considered it a good trade for survival and peace of mind."

Wanda Null; diagnosed in 1986 at the age of 41; librarian

"My husband has been wonderful. He says he doesn't even see the scars that go across my breasts. They are there and probably always will be, but he is just grateful I am here to help raise our children."

Tresa Johnson; diagnosed in 1999 at the age of 23; PA

"From the day of my diagnosis, I vowed that I would take each step to survival one step at a time. After each step comes a big reward. I try to think of fun things I can do with my husband that remind us we have so much more living to do. Just five days after my lumpectomy, we took a week's holiday abroad. It was the best thing we could have done! Although I was recovering from the operation and was a little sore, I was living life! After chemo, there will be another trip before radiotherapy. Having this to look forward to really helps."

Helen Lawlor; diagnosed in 2000 at the age of 43; medical communications operative

Sweet Single

"After the operation, I was able to make fun of myself, telling my brother that I went in for a breast reduction and they made a mistake and took it all!"
Jacqueline Durant; diagnosed in 1994 at the age of 68; retired

"I was determined that if I was going to give up a breast, I was going to get something out of it. So, not only did I ask my plastic surgeon to make my other breast match the new one, I asked her to fix my earlobes, so that I could wear pierced ear-rings again!"
Rosamary Amiet; diagnosed in 2000 at the age of 48; programme manager

"My boyfriend was with me when the doctor told me I had breast cancer. He said that all he heard was 'It's curable' and that was enough for him. I sometimes talk about my different breast in front of others, and he says, 'Doesn't bother me. I always preferred the other one, anyway.' "
Sharon Daniels; diagnosed in 2000 at the age of 49; hairdresser, wig shop owner

"I don't care if other women see me undressing with only one breast. I'm just thankful to be alive!"
Billie Loop; diagnosed in 1997 at the age of 63; housewife

"To destroy a bosom is a form of mental rape.
Were I younger and had life ahead
I would resent the need that made it necessary
To invade my person.
However, cancer forces reality.
Medical skill keeps me alive.
My gratitude bows to surgeons.
Forgiveness is my pride."
Barbara M. Wells; diagnosed in 1999 at the age of 78; mother, writer

"This is for anyone who is contemplating having reconstruction surgery after a mastectomy. As the Nike ad says, 'Just do it!' Before my surgery, I didn't consider reconstruction. For two and a half years, I wore a special bra with my prosthesis, and I knew that many women were doing the same thing. But eventually the idea of

replacing my 'flat' side with a 'bump' began to appeal to me more and more. I was only in my early fifties and had decided that there was no reason why I would not live a normal lifespan. So I had an implant inserted and later had a nipple areola reconstruction. After my experience, I would recommend reconstruction for anyone who may be wondering if it is worth the surgery. Vanity is not the issue here, but there is nothing like being able to dress without special 'equipment'. Life gets better and better each day!"
Gail Blackmer; diagnosed in 1997 at the age of 50; teacher's assistant

"The upside to having reconstructive surgery is that your breast will never sag!"
Debby Whittet; diagnosed in 1996 at the age of 43; housewife, part-time library worker

"I waited 18 months before I had the courage to go for reconstructive surgery, and then I had a TRAM-flap reconstruction. It was a rough operation, worse actually than the mastectomy, but well worth it. I feel much better than when I was wearing a prosthesis. And I got a tummy tuck in the process!"
Rebecca Clarkson; diagnosed in 1997 at the age of 45; road transport worker

"I decided to have reconstruction for balance. I only had one breast removed and didn't want to be lopsided. I thought briefly about a prosthesis, but decided I wanted something more permanent. I had this vision of coming back from holiday having left it in the room. I imagined having to call the hotel and ask if anyone had found a breast in room 123."
Val Long; diagnosed in 1999 at the age of 47; administrative assistant

"It really helped me to go into hospital with two breasts and come home with two breasts. I had reconstruction that used my own muscle and tissue. I'm very happy with the results. My breast looks normal again, and this makes me feel complete."
Gwen Loverink; diagnosed in 1994 at the age of 34; police dispatcher

"When I was diagnosed with breast cancer, I did not panic. I simply made up my mind to do everything I could to beat it. I had a mastectomy and reconstruction, and this made me feel whole again. It has been more than two years now, and I am healthy

and happy."
Ann Gordon; diagnosed in 1998 at the age of 73; retired business
executive

Two's a Couple

"Both of my breasts had been cystic, and I'd had questionable lumps removed from both over many years. So it made sense to me to stop living with the emotional roller-coaster and have both breasts removed in a single operation. It is a wonderful feeling to be finished with that part of my life."
Carol Hattler; diagnosed in 1999 at the age of 65; retired nurse

"Waiting for breast cancer to arrive for many years provided me with the opportunity to decide what I would do about it. My sister Adelaide was diagnosed with breast cancer 20 years before I was and my sister Elizabeth two years before I was. Although I only had cancer in one breast, I had both removed. Being pragmatic, I never liked wearing a bra, and I couldn't imagine always being unbalanced. Now I can run like I did when I was ten years old."
Cleves Daniels Weber; diagnosed in 1999 at the age of 60; owner,
metaphysical bookshop

"I was diagnosed at 35. I was fortunate enough to have doctors who caught the disease early, but when it came to treatment, I told them I wanted a double mastectomy. I had been a 44DD for most of my life, and being free of the cancer seemed to be a good trade-off. I walked around the month after my surgery wearing a T-shirt, and I felt like a little kid. I wouldn't say that I have been worry free, especially being in my late thirties and dealing with my boyfriend, but guess what? We both appreciate the fact that I am here."
Marian Anne Miziorko; diagnosed in 1995 at the age of 35; tax inspector

"When it came to reconstruction, I only went for a small bulge so that I wouldn't be so flat. Now, when I look at my chest, I think that I look like a female athlete. I do not miss my old lopsided breasts, and I love not having to wear bras. I feel alive and more feminine. I feel free!"
Carol Hattler; diagnosed in 1999 at the age of 65; retired nurse

"Twelve years ago, I had breast cancer in both breasts. I had recon-

struction and loved it. I had always been a D-cup, so surgery was my
salvation – getting rid of those *big* breasts!"
Mary Ann Lee; diagnosed in 1988 at the age of 46; tax collector

"I have to say that in spite of everything I went through, I did get
beautiful breasts."
Tobi Stelzer; diagnosed in 1997 at the age of 40; teacher

"The first time I saw my sister-in-law after her reconstructive
surgery (after a double mastectomy at the age of 27), I found I was
trying very hard not to glance down at her chest. But finally, I
couldn't contain myself any longer and admitted this . . . to which
Barbra replied, 'Here,' as she proudly opened her jacket to reveal
a tight sweater through which I could see the shape of her breasts.
'They're great, aren't they?' And I have to admit they *were* great!"
Wendy Page; sister-in-law of Barbra Marcus Kolton

"The thing that helped me get over being self-conscious was having
reconstruction. It was a big boost to my morale. After it was completed, I went out and bought a sexy bra and suspenders. I wore
them for my husband on our 25th wedding anniversary."
Polly Briggs; diagnosed in 1987 at the age of 41; secretary

"The upside of my reconstruction was that after years of suffering
gravity's pull, I could now go without a bra."
Barbara Moro; diagnosed in 1999 at the age of 57; legal secretary

Who Needs Breasts!

"For those who may wonder whether everyone has reconstruction,
I did not, and I have never regretted it. I still feel feminine and
sexy. Occasionally I may mention to my husband that perhaps I
should have at least thought about reconstruction, and he
responds, 'Why?' For several years I would look in the mirror after
bathing and wonder when the scar and/or the absence of a breast
would bother me. In nine years it never has. The only thing the
scar does is remind me how lucky I am."
Jane Vaughan; diagnosed in 1991 at the age of 53; writer

"I was diagnosed in 1993 and had a modified radical mastectomy.
After two and a half years, I finished with my yearning for recon-

struction by deciding against it and instead getting a tattoo etched on my mastectomy side. It is a very tasteful scene of a humming-bird sipping nectar from a rose-vine type of plant, and a monarch butterfly is hovering close by. I've been able to display my tattoo to a diverse audience, and it has proven therapeutic for the viewer as well as for me."
Kathy Kirkley; diagnosed in 1993 at the age of 40; nurse, mother, wife

"I don't have any breasts and I don't care. I don't have to wear a bra and I can jog without pain. I know that people love me for what's on the inside, not for my physical appearance."
Cindy Bird; diagnosed in 1998 at the age of 39; personnel officer

"I have a very positive outlook in life. So when all the bandages were taken off, I said, 'Sue, be strong with the help of God. When you look into the mirror, you now have one smiley and one hung low, but you are alive.' "
Suzanne Almond; diagnosed in 1996 at the age of 60; secretary

"Not long after my surgery, my partner and I attended a women's retreat. During the course of the weekend, many women took their clothes off and jumped into the swimming pool. Of all the differ-ent body shapes, I noticed two women, one who had a single mas-tectomy and the other a bilateral. And there I stood trying to muster enough courage to do the same. I was waiting for the sun to disappear or some act of Mother Nature that would force all these women out of the pool. Heather was already in the pool waiting for me. Slowly, I undressed and entered the pool. Within minutes the tears started to roll down my cheeks. No one stared, no one turned away so as not to see my bare chest. It was okay even without a cou-ple of body parts."
Carol Snyder; diagnosed in 1992 at the age of 47; special needs teacher

"I had several male friends, colleagues, who were so supportive that it brought tears to my eyes. One even went to counselling so that he could help me. He was very comfortable discussing any-thing and everything, a true and rare friend. Thus far, the men I've told about my mastectomy have shrugged, telling me that I'm more than the sum of one body part. Frankly, I'm surprised, given how our society places an enormous value on breasts. But I'm not

complaining. Perhaps men are somewhat enlightened after all."
Marti Devich; diagnosed in 1980 at the age of 34; saleswoman, business owner, writer

". . . Mastectomy.
What a horrible word.
An ending – the removal of something so essential to womanhood.
But is it?
No, I think not.
Womanhood stems from our hearts and minds.
If necessary, I would sacrifice my breast to preserve my life."
Mary Platt; diagnosed in 1998 at the age of 47; radiology supervisor

3 • Radiotherapy

Soaking Up the Rays

W hen I learned that my treatment plan called for 30 sessions of radiotherapy – five sessions a week for six weeks – I was dismayed. This would mean driving 45 minutes each way, to the hospital and back, every day. Forget cancer, city traffic is stressful to me. Besides, I was in the middle of writing a book, which typically requires my uninterrupted concentration from eight in the morning until six at night. Radiotherapy would take a two-hour chunk out of that time, day after day.

How to turn that into a plus? I could request an early morning or late afternoon session, but those slots were in demand by women who held jobs with less flexible hours than mine. I had the luxury of being my own boss. Taking that in its broadest sense, I simply shifted my thinking.

I planned my sessions for two in the afternoon. I worked at my computer until I had to leave, then used the driving time not to feel stressed about traffic or cancer but to mull over what I'd written, make changes on a tape recorder and plot what I would write when I got home. Know what? There wasn't the slightest blip in my productivity during that entire six-week span.

With a few exceptions when my sons were home on holiday and drove me in, or when my husband met me at the hospital, or when

33

a friend insisted on coming, I went to radiotherapy alone. Just like finishing on the weight machine after getting the phone call that said I had *it*, this meant a lot to me. I've always been independent, have always hated imposing on people. Driving myself to daily treatments was consistent with this, particularly since the radiotherapy itself took no time at all. It was also another reminder to myself, and to my husband, my sons and the few friends who knew, that I was healthy, strong, and as good as ever.

Having experienced radiotherapy, I felt particularly strongly about the need for a chapter on it in *UPLIFT*. When I was told not to use deodorant, for example, I had no idea what to use in its place. The doctors shrugged, as did the radiotherapists. They didn't know. But survivors do.

Various submissions gave various reasons why traditional deodorants are banned during radiation. After reading one explanation too many, I sent a frantic e-mail to a friend whose husband is a radiotherapist. As he explained it, the high density of trace metals in traditional deodorants can sensitise the skin, making it more likely to become irritated and even burnt. Doctors believe that these metals seep into the skin so that they cannot be completely washed off before daily treatments. Hence the ban.

A final word, while I have your attention. Tattoos. Typically, these are applied during the planning session before the start of radiotherapy. They take seconds to apply and hurt only as much as an elastic band might if it were snapped against the skin. I won't explain their purpose, since Deb Haney has explained it so well in the section on tattoos. Suffice it to say that most women don't mind them at all, which I think is the best way to be. They aren't obtrusive. As many women point out, they are a badge of courage – a reminder that you've had something and been cured. In that, they serve a positive purpose.

I wish I could be as accepting as these women. But I'm not.

Oh, getting those tattoos was a piece of cake – though I have to say that I hadn't realised, until mere minutes before mine were applied, that they were part of the process. No one had told me that, and I was irked. But there were two other things that bothered me more.

First, I had always wanted a tattoo but hadn't had the courage to get one. Nice girls didn't do that, or so the story went; classy women didn't do it either. But suddenly it seemed unfair that I didn't have the tattoo I wanted, while I *did* have ones that I didn't want.

Second, one of the seven little blue dots that had been permanently inked into my skin was smack in the middle of my chest. I only had to wear a scoop neckline, and there it was, like the mark of Cain. Please know that I wasn't embarrassed to have people see it – and even if I was, no one ever noticed mine, and I do wear my share of scoop necklines. That dot might have easily passed as a birthmark. It was truly tiny.

The problem was me. I was dealing with breast cancer by doing everything medically that I could while keeping the rest of my life the same as ever – but there it was, that tattoo, staring back at me in the mirror every day, reminding me of what I'd had.

But I knew what I'd had – "had" being the operative word. The cancer had gone; I wanted the tattoo to go, too. It had served its purpose. I didn't see why I needed to keep it.

So I acted. First, I made an appointment at a laser centre that advertised tattoo removal. It turned out that the removal of those tiny blue dots took mere seconds each. When I pulled out my wallet to pay, the doctor said, "No charge. You didn't ask for those tattoos. You shouldn't have to pay to have them removed."

Second, I got my own tattoo – one that I wanted – one that I see in the mirror every day and have never yet regretted. Nope. I'm not telling what it is or where, only that it brings great pleasure to my husband and me.

Making It Easier

"Different family members and friends went with me for my radiotherapy treatments. We always went out for breakfast afterwards."
Sharon Erbe; diagnosed in 1999 at the age of 54; nursing teacher

"For my first radiotherapy treatments, I had to travel a long way each day. We lived in a rural area and our friends and neighbours got together without my knowledge and scheduled one of them to drive me each day so that my husband could continue to work. I never knew who would drive up to take me until whoever it was arrived."
Kathleen Griffith; diagnosed in 1976 at the age of 42; bookkeeper

"I continued to work during my treatments, but I took off every Friday, when I had either treatment or blood testing. When it came time for radiotherapy, I shortened my working day so that I could have treatment and be home before the kids got off the bus."
Deborah J. P. Schur; diagnosed in 1994 at the age of 43; sales rep

"Each day that I went for a treatment, there was a small anonymous gift waiting for me at my place at the kitchen table. The gifts were placed after I retired at night and before I arose at 6 a.m. After about three weeks, I realised that there was a let-down feeling on Saturdays and Sundays because there was no gift. These were really little things like a fancy pencil or a small notebook, but they lifted my spirits. It was not until after all the treatments that I was told that one daughter had the idea and started the 'gift bag' to have something for another daughter to put out each night."
Lela Quimby; diagnosed in 1985 at the age of 56; retired teacher

"I love lattes and looked forward to the treat every day after radiotherapy."
Marge Fuller; diagnosed in 1994 at the age of 63; education authority officer, retired

"During radiotherpy, I visualised myself on a beach under the healing light of the sun. I felt strength moving through me. My treatments took place in February. My family held an *indoor beach party* to celebrate."
Sharon Erbe; diagnosed in 1999 at the age of 54; nursing teacher

"In the midst of radiotherapy, my wonderful husband, who is my rock, kidnapped me one Friday and took me to a hotel for a romantic weekend away just for us. It helped me to remember that I am a woman who is loved."
Nancie Watson; diagnosed in 1995 at the age of 50; social worker

Tattoos

"The reason you get tattooed is that, with permanent marks to align the machines on, they can treat the exact same area each day. But I had never heard about the tattoos before radiotherapy, and my mind raced off in all directions. I pictured myself with a *huge*

black domino shape tattooed on one side of my chest – big round black dots that would be with me for ever, like giant cards out of *Alice in Wonderland* or a funky biker tattoo. My fear stayed with me until the day I went in for orientation and tattooing at the radio-therapy centre. Much to my relief, the radiotherapist was a sensitive young girl and the tattoos she made were no larger than tiny pinpricks."
Deb Haney; diagnosed in 1996 at the age of 48; administrative assistant, artist

"I had always said that when I turned 40, I would get a tattoo, but I chickened out. Well, hey, I did get my tattoos. I thought that was pretty good."
Dee Pobjoy; diagnosed in 1999 at the age of 41; sales clerk

"I recently read of some women who want to get their radiotherapy tattoos removed. I say, 'No way!' These are a symbol of all I've been through and have overcome."
Fran Hegarty; diagnosed in 2000 at the age of 47; librarian

"I hate my tattoos. I notice them every day and they remind me that I have had breast cancer. But they also remind me that I am very lucky and I am a survivor."
Suzanne Pollock; diagnosed in 1995 at the age of 50; stationer

"What to do with my tattoos? I have three down the centre of my chest. My friend says I should make the top one into a dolphin diving down into my breast."
Pam Waddell; diagnosed in 1998 at the age of 38; writer, teacher's assistant

"I consider my tattoos badges of honour. I have survived. No one has ever asked me what they are – but should anyone ever do that, I would ask if they have had a mammogram this year."
Nancie Watson; diagnosed in 1995 at the age of 50; social worker

"I have a suggestion. Instead of the black tattoo dots, why not use a small rose or a butterfly? At least then people wouldn't think you had a spot of dirt on your neck."
Kathleen Griffith; diagnosed in 1976 at the age of 42; bookkeeper

"My radiotherapist didn't use tattoos. Instead, I got marked up daily with a purple marker. On my days off from therapy, I had to be careful not to wash off the marks or smear them off with the skin creams I used to condition my skin. I ended up wearing a man's T-shirt under my clothing to protect it from being ruined."
Sharon Irons Strempski; diagnosed in 1997 at the age of 52; nurse

"I bought inexpensive sports bras without underwires for radiation. The indelible ink that they use to mark your tattoos ruins good bras, and, at the end, when your skin is sore, the lack of underwires helped. I still wear bras without underwires."
Suzanne Pollock; diagnosed in 1995 at the age of 50; stationer

"I brought black bras and a camisole, so that marks painted on me for radiotherapy would not destroy good clothes."
Pauline Hughes; diagnosed in 1997 at the age of 61; retired nurse

Nuts and Bolts

"Usually, as I lay in the radiotherapy room, watching the lights of the equipment, I would be visualising a good sparkling 'rain' coming into my body, washing its way through, with the 'bad' cells flowing out through my feet and far, far away. Visualisation will speed up the healing, removing the stress of the moment and bringing you peace!"
Deb Haney; diagnosed in 1996 at the age of 48; administrative assistant, artist

"Early in radiotherapy, the sound of the machine released the floodgate of fear I was trying to hold back. Knowing I could not get through the radiotherapy crying, I began talking to friends who were not there . . . or singing. These sounds diverted my thoughts and enabled me to put the sound of the radiotherapy machine in the background."
Jeanne Sturdevant; diagnosed in 1990 at the age of 45; artist

"Radiotherapy is tiring. When I asked why, I was told that since the treatment was killing cells, the good cells have to work overtime. That makes sense to me."
Sharon Daniels; diagnosed in 2000 at the age of 49; hairdresser, wig shop owner

"While I was having radiotherapy, a friend of mine suggested having a glass of red wine once a day to keep my blood up. It was wonderful and worked beautifully. Also, a small glass of sherry about half an hour before meals helped the appetite."
Barbara C. Sumner; diagnosed in 1982 at the age of 59; housewife

"Talking and opening up to others in the radiotherapy waiting room was very important. I made a firm friend there. We all felt sorry for one woman who resisted passing the time of day with anyone. Holding back completely is so harmful. Everyone needs the concern and compassion of those who are going through what they are."
Sheila Roper; diagnosed in 1995 at the age of 57; housewife

Deodorant

"I put pure cornstarch in a beautiful shaker (for powdered sugar really) and used that for deodorant under the affected arm."
Suzanne Pollock; diagnosed in 1995 at the age of 50; stationer

"My mother's radiologist recommended that she use unscented Dove soap while she was undergoing radiotherapy."
Barbara Keiler; daughter of survivor

"One deodorant to use that contains no aluminium salts is something called Pit Rok, a 100 gram stick of 100 per cent natural mineral salts. You simply wet the stick and rub it on."
Gracie Schwingel; diagnosed in 1998 at the age of 51; secretary

"When you go for radiation, take a zip-up bag with a moist flannel and a shaker of pure cornstarch. Use them in the changing room after treatment."
Rayna Ragonetti; diagnosed in 1993 at the age of 52; executive

"I was afraid of getting an infection in the arm where the few lymph nodes were removed. So I was very careful and did not shave under my arms or use deodorant for a while. I washed the area several times a day. When healed, I carefully shaved and used a baking soda-based deodorant."
Carol Hattler; diagnosed in 1999 at the age of 65; retired nurse

Too Much Sun . . .

"Those clear 100 per cent aloe vera gels are very soothing for skin burnt from the radiotherapy."
Sharon Irons Strempski; diagnosed in 1997 at the age of 52; nurse

"I used liquid vitamin E on my skin to help the dryness."
Therese Gunty; diagnosed in 1997 at the age of 70; housewife

"When I was going through radiotherapy, my aloe vera plant was my best friend. Every morning I broke off a leaf, put it in my little Tupperware container and when I finished that day's treatment, I slit the leaf open and rubbed it over the radiotherapy site. Most of the healthcare professionals laughed. They told me to wait until I had skin symptoms. My reply was, "When do you put sunscreen on . . . before you go out in the sun, or after you get sunburnt?" I am happy to report that I had no skin reaction at all! And, if you want to hear something spooky, after the plant had been used 32 times, just when my radiotherapy was over, she stopped growing! Guess she thought her work was done! I have since given friends aloe vera plants when they are undergoing radiotherapy, and no one has complained. I even passed along the Tupperware container to a friend when she was newly diagnosed, as apparently it had such good vibes."
Sheilah Musselman; diagnosed in 1997 at the age of 56; nurse

"During my radiotherapy, I used mild Dove soap. A week after my last treatment, I got really burnt and peeled. I smothered 100 per cent (clear) aloe vera gel on my breast and put a medicinal pad over it so it did not stick to my clothes. It cleared up in a week."
Candice Jaeger; diagnosed in 2000 at the age of 24; wife and mother

"My breast started to shrink! Fourteen months after my radiotherapy was complete, my affected breast suddenly looked markedly smaller than the other one. I was sure that it would shrink to just a nipple! The truth is that it can take about that long for the fluid to be reabsorbed post-operatively. Yeah, that breast will be smaller . . . but I can live with it!"
Donna Barnett; diagnosed in 1999 at the age of 40; nurse

"When I had radiotherapy, I used pure aloe vera gel on the area that got burnt. Because the area under my arm was sensitive and the edge of my bra rubbed it, I sewed a small piece of new blanket material over the offending edge. When the last few treatments zeroed in on the area around my nipple, where the cancer had been, I coated a square of gauze with petroleum jelly and placed it there after each treatment. That brought much relief."

Lela Quimby, diagnosed in 1985 at the age of 56; retired teacher

Comfort Clothes

"During radiotherapy, when your skin is most sensitive, wear over-sized white cotton T-shirts cut off at the waist, and cut the sleeves out. Then turn them inside out so the seams do not rub."

Caroline C. Hudnall; diagnosed in 1992 at the age of 55; retired court official; Montana

"Because I could not wear a bra and had to have very soft cotton next to my skin, I purchased matching cotton teddies and sexy briefs. What a boost!"

Nancie Watson; diagnosed in 1995 at the age of 50; social worker

"I wore soft clothes like polar fleece almost constantly. Also, treatment areas can be pretty chilly, so taking a soft shawl with you can be a comfort."

Christine Foutris; diagnosed in 1999 at the age of 49; teacher

"Buy soft cotton vests. They will help after the operation, since your skin will be sensitive, and provide a place to attach drainage tubes."

Alexandra Koffman; diagnosed in 1996 at the age of 40; nurse

"Feel like a kid again. Wear cotton bras with no underwiring during radiotherapy. Wear T-shirts in bright colours with comical characters, such as Tweety Pie. I bought a wraparound shirt in a stretch material that I could wear during radiotherapy. This saved time undressing and dressing. I had very early morning appointments, then went directly to my office from the hospital."

Ellen Beth Simon; diagnosed in 1998 at the age of 41; lawyer

"As for favourite clothing during treatment, I bought a two-piece

velvet-velour lounge suit that is as comfortable as a pair of pyjamas and elegant enough for entertaining visitors. It is also very soft against my skin."
Carrie Drake; diagnosed in 1998 at the age of 42; administrative assistant

"During radiotherapy, breast tissue can become very tender. A simple support garment can be made by using 'tube' material, which can be purchased at most drapery shops. This material comes in a wide variety of colours. Measure enough to reach just past your waist. Stitch ¼ inch of elastic to the top, zigzag-stitch the bottom to prevent the fabric from unravelling, and this makes a most comfortable strapless bra that can be used by both large- and small-breasted women. It goes on easily, comes off easily, does not bind sensitive shoulders, and can be washed and dried using regular washing and drying cycles. It certainly provides non-binding relief to sensitive skin areas."
Florence Wade; diagnosed in 1999 at the age of 63; retired schoolteacher and property manager

Stories

"When my doctor advised me to have radiotherapy, I told him that I didn't want to. He told me that it would increase my survival rate, and still I said no. With this, he looked me straight in the eye and said, 'Then I'd advise you to go over to Chernobyl in the Ukraine and stand in the middle of the town with all that radioactive material that leaked from the reactor!' I burst out laughing at such a ridiculous picture. Then I decided that radiotherapy wouldn't be so bad after all if I did it the American way. At another point, this same doctor snapped me out of a dark mood by saying, 'Brenda, you are going to die, but not from this.' That was in 1986."
Brenda M. Kraft; diagnosed in 1986 at the age of 60; retired schoolteacher

"When I learned that I would have 35 days of radiotherapy, I wrote to the 35 most important women in my life and asked them to send T-shirts in lieu of flowers. The shirts, I explained, would be helpful in eliminating the minutia in my life – like "Whatever shall I wear to radiotherapy for 35 days?" Over 60 shirts arrived – some new, some old and familiar. I felt closer to these friends in their shirts, and they knew that they had done something for me that we would both remember. Someone else's cotton shirt against your skin brings them close to your heart."

Betsy Ellis Bowles; diagnosed in 2000 at the age of 57; private mortgage banker

"Sometimes I would lie there wondering how the radiotherapist felt, knowing they were helping people heal but also causing damage in the process. Since it was Christmas, I wanted to do something to lighten the atmosphere. So I got an art book from the library and copied a large photo of one of the beautiful Roman lady statues with her arm up over her head and her bare breast hanging out of her tunic – a pose that I and dozens of others assumed every day. I made a Christmas card, almost like a small poster, that said, 'Happy Christmas – to a great gang to "hang out" with.' The next time I went in for treatment, it was hanging on the wall in the cubicle where the radiotherapist stood!"

Deb Haney; diagnosed in 1996 at the age of 48; administrative assistant, artist

"What do we need from our carers and significant others? I needed to be heard in a holistic way. I needed my doctor to acknowledge my mental needs as well as my medical ones. My oncologist stood still and listened; it was an amazing gift."

Jeanne Sturdevant; diagnosed in 1990 at the age of 45; artist

"I argued with the radiologist every time I had my yearly mammogram because they would charge full price, though I had only one breast. I tried different hospitals and clinics and found the same thing. I won my fight when one hospital finally sent me a letter saying that they would never again charge a patient with only one breast for a bilateral test. I always have my mammogram there now."

Earlene Smith; diagnosed in 1985 at the age of 52; part-time postal worker

"When my friend started her 35 radiotherapy treatments, I made a big calendar, and we counted down the seven weeks. When it was over, we celebrated with a dinner. I sent her flowers with a card that read, 'Congratulations to a survivor. You did it!' "

Grace Trocco; friend of two survivors

4 • Chemo and Hair

Mane Matters

Losing her hair is every woman's fear. You don't have to face chemotherapy to know this. Take a look at any magazine. Right up there with skin-and-bones in the beauty department is hair. There are products promoting healthy hair, swingy hair, shiny hair and thick hair. There are ones promoting curls, ones that make hair straight and sleek, ones that colour it here and there, or all over. Okay. So you can avoid magazines. But you have to buy food at the supermarket, and you can find haircare products there, too. Walk outside and there's the side of a bus emblazoned with a gorgeous face surrounded by a riot of wonderful hair. It doesn't have to be long hair. It can be short, but it's always shiny and sexy.

So, what if you don't *have* hair? What then? How do you feel? How do those around you feel? How do you go out without thinking that everyone is staring at you? How do you maintain a semblance of femininity?

The devastation of losing hair to chemotherapy is a major issue for women. This came through loud and clear in the earliest submissions to *UPLIFT*. In fact, the subject generated enough response to earn a chapter of its own.

Now, everything in *UPLIFT* is meant to be upbeat. By way of setting the scene, though, I'd like to quote Lori Bartz. Lori was diagnosed in 2000 at the age of 41. She had sent an early submission, which opened, "It seems weird to say that breast cancer could in any way improve my life, but it has." Later, though, she sent another note. I share this one with you in part because I sense that it echoes what many of you are feeling, in part because the people around us need to know that as upbeat as we are, we sometimes have to moan, and in part because it illustrates one woman's ability to feel lousy but still rebound.

"The worst part of this entire experience," Lori wrote, "is losing my hair. I *hate* wigs, though I have had many, many compliments, some from people who don't know it's a wig. The chemotherapy would be so much easier if I had my own hair. I appreciate that the drugs are killing my cancer, but I still want my hair. I can finally look at my head, but it still seriously upsets me. I feel selfish that this 'hair issue' is so important to me. I can hide the mastectomy, but it's not so easy to hide a bald head. Thanks for the opportunity to moan about this issue."

You're welcome, Lori. I'd bet that women all over the place are nodding in agreement – and it isn't that researchers aren't working their tails off to find chemo drugs that don't cause hair loss. I believe that there are already some possibilities, though many more trials are needed before those drugs become widely used. In the meantime, we're stuck with bald heads. But that's not the end of the world.

Listen to Deborah Schur, a sales rep, who was diagnosed in 1994 at the age of 43. She wrote, "I remember saying to one of the men I work with that if I lost all my hair, I would be ugly. His reply was that even without hair, I would be beautiful. He also reminded me, sternly and realistically, that my hair would grow back."

A final word from Lori again, who concluded her note this way. "Thank God for my husband. He says I look 'cute' with no hair, hence the saying 'Love is blind'."

Take "love" in its broadest sense, and you have the heart of this chapter.

Losing It

"Don't let the drugs call the shots. When your hair first starts to fall out, cut it all off. You now have control. And remember, the sooner it falls out, the sooner it grows back!"
Susan Schultz; diagnosed in 1990 at the age of 41; special needs assistant

"My friend Meg came to see me with her hair cut shorter and shorter each time. One day when she came over, she smiled and took off her hat. She had shaved her head. Right behind her came her husband, who whipped off his hat to show he had shaved *his* head, too. What a team!"
Betty Schulte; friend of a survivor

"My 27-year-old daughter Karen came to visit at the time when my hair was coming out daily in clumps. I kept saying to her that I just wished it would all fall out and be done with it. Taking my hand, she led me into the bathroom, and we shaved my head. It was a great moment. She finally felt there was something she could do to help, and I realised that I wasn't alone."
Carol Englund; diagnosed in 1994 at the age of 58; retired administrative assistant

"I'll never forget the day we shaved my head. My best friend, Susan, who normally styles my hair, insisted on doing it. My son Mike, who always has a smart remark, took one look at me and asked Susan how much she charged for that haircut! Then when my other son, Matt, approached me, we could see the shock. So Susan said, 'Look at this cute little baldini.' From that day on, Matt kissed my bald head every single day and asked how his cute little baldini was. I'll never forget it. He made my day!"
Anita Leuzzi; diagnosed in 1997 at the age of 45; legal secretary

"I had a haircutting party to which I invited 15 of my friends. They took turns chopping off sections of my long hair and tying them with pink ribbons. The party was a way for me to feel more in control of the situation. It also involved my friends in the process, so that they didn't feel as helpless."
Asha Mevlana; diagnosed in 1999 at the age of 24; musician

"When my extremely thick hair began falling out fast and furious, leaving unsightly bald spots, my husband shaved my head. That reduced the 'fallout' considerably but left me with an itchy, irritated scalp. What helped me most was taking long, hot showers every morning and night (all that water rushing over my shaved head felt good!), then rubbing vitamin E oil all over the scalp. I put a towel over my pillow at night so I didn't leak oil on to the pillowcase. My scalp was healthier and less itchy the very next day. Any extra oil can be rubbed on to the scar tissue on the breast, which will help it heal faster."

Margaret Blair; diagnosed in 2000 at the age of 49; writer

"When my hair started falling out, I didn't know what to expect. Would it all come out at once? What does a 44-year-old woman look like with no hair? I sat outside and pulled and pulled until I couldn't pull any more. It took me longer to get up enough nerve to look in the mirror than to do all the pulling. Then, because I looked like Bozo the Clown on a really bad hair day, I went to the beautician's, where they shaved my head. But what about all those little stubs that kept falling out? My solution? Parcel tape. I wrapped this around my hand and kept applying it until my head was as smooth as a pool ball."

Denise Judy; diagnosed in 1999 at the age of 43; sign language specialist

"When I reached the point where I could pull my hair out in clumps, I asked my partner to accompany me to a local nature sanctuary. We went to one of my favourite meadows, where the grasses and wildflowers grow tall and the forest surrounded us. I pulled out handfuls of hair and scattered it in the wind, hoping the birds and mice would use it to make warm, soft nests. For me, this simple spiritual act transformed the trauma of chemo-induced hair loss into a connection with the earth and with life."

Dorian Solot; diagnosed in 2000 at the age of 26

"My hair started falling out after my first treatment. I got tired of waking up with hair all over my pillowcase and seeing lost hair going down the plughole. I decided to take matters into my own hands. My fabulous hairdresser Lori decided to take a day off work and drive me to an upmarket wig salon that came highly recommended. Well, I don't know how many of these salons you have ever visited, but this was my first experience. They ushered us into a private room complete with salon chair mirrors and wig products galore. Lori put one wig on after another . . . nothing felt right. Too dark, too light, too curly, too itchy. We then started trying on the hats . . . now we were having some fun! I realised that wigs were not for me and that wigs or hats, my head would still be bald! We left the salon that day with a few hats and drove home hatching another plan. The next evening with a glass of wine in my hand and my husband standing nervously outside the door of Lori's hairdressing salon, she proceeded to shave my head. She cried as she did it, but said that I had courage. For me, taking matters into my own hands was important. That day, I also learned that a good hairdresser does not just cut hair."

Cindy Fiedler; diagnosed in 1998 at the age of 40; registered nurse, mother

"The worst was when I started losing my hair, but when that happened, at the suggestion of my hairdresser, I had my head shaved. I put on a wig immediately, and it made it much easier. When my hair started to grow back, it was like peach fuzz, so I felt that I was in fashion! When it started getting long, I could tell it was thicker than it had been, and soft as a baby's."

Barbara Moro; diagnosed in 1999 at the age of 57; legal secretary

"If you're going to lose your hair, cut it short before you begin the therapy. Long hair can clog sink and bath plugholes when it falls out. Who needs a plumbing hassle when you're undergoing chemo?"

Barbara Keiler; daughter of a survivor

"Early on after my neighbour was diagnosed, she chose to shave her head rather than watch her very long, thick, plaited hair fall out clumps at a time. As she is a statuesque dark-skinned lady, it was actually quite becoming."

Nancy Summersong; friend of a survivor

"When my hair started falling out, I had my husband shave it off. As horrifying as that was, I felt it was better to have it off quickly, than have a mess coming out in your hands, comb and brush, on your pillow, and so forth."

Rhonda Sorrell; diagnosed in 1998 at the age of 43; special needs teacher

"My hair started to fall out on 1st April. Yes, April Fool's Day. Some joke! People told me that it was a good sign, that it meant the chemotherapy had started working. I don't know if that's true or not, but it did help. At first I cried a little, but then I took control. I decided that looking at my thinning hair every day would be more difficult than looking at a bald head. So I called my hairdresser and had the remainder of my hair buzzed off. I felt much better. The thinning hair represented what the disease could do to my body. My buzzed head represented strength and control. I was in charge."

Val Long; diagnosed in 1999 at the age of 47; administrative assistant

"When I knew I would lose my hair, I cut it short into a style that I wasn't particularly crazy about. It wasn't so hard to lose a 'bad' short hairstyle as it would have been to lose my longer hair. I have to say that I found it fascinating to just run my fingers through my hair and come away with a handful. I thought that if the drugs are powerful enough to take my hair, what a job they must be doing on those cancer cells! When it got to the point where there wasn't much hair left, I took some scissors and cut it down to the scalp. That much I had control over!"

Gwen Loverink; diagnosed in 1994 at the age of 34; police dispatcher

"I was strangely intrigued by the thought of my hair falling out. Would I just wake up bald one morning, or would it come out gradually for days? I was told to expect it to fall out between Days 14 and 22 following my first treatment, so every day beginning on about Day 10, I'd wake up, tug on my hair, and assure myself that it was still firmly attached to my head. On Day 16, we had an unusually warm March day, and I decided to enjoy the fresh air as I drove along the road. Bad idea! I almost choked to death with all the hair flying around the car. Since I hadn't been losing it up until that point, at first I couldn't decide what it was that kept blowing into my mouth. When I realised it was my hair, I pulled the car over to the side of the road to inspect my head in the mirror. There was no noticeable change yet, but I knew the process had begun. I soon learned that there's nothing gradual at all about the hair-falling-out phase. It is just not fun to vacuum your own hair from the bathroom floor or change the sheets and pillowcases as soon as you get up in the morning. By Day 19, I was more than ready for the 'buzz party' that my husband and I had planned. We went out the back of the house, and he lovingly and silently buzzed my head. When he was finished, we collected all the hair and left a pile for the birds that were nesting in the eaves. For some reason, that pleased me. When we were back in the house, my husband gave me a big hug and assured me that I looked 'just great'. I found that hard to believe, since I didn't look so terrific *with* hair, but I appreciated the sentiment. It didn't take me long to put the whole hair issue into perspective. Okay, I was an overweight, middle-aged, fuzzy-headed woman. I was also on the road to recovery from a life-threatening illness, and I began to view my hair loss as a testimony to this struggle – sort of like a 'badge of courage'."

Nancy Lane; diagnosed in 2000 at the age of 53; teacher

"I cut Judi's hair all off yesterday. She rang up, wondering if I would be comfortable enough to do it, then arranging a time. She appeared around noon, beach towel and kitchen scissors in hand. Not the tools of a trained hairdresser to be sure, but the best we could come up with. We spread the towel on the kitchen floor, put a chair on the towel, snapped a 'before' picture, and she sat down. I picked up her short blonde waves and cut them off. They went into the bin in handfuls, the blonde sun-bleached top, then the brown locks from underneath. We saved a handful, a mixture of both colours, in a plastic bag for posterity. Judi is my good friend who shares my name and neighbourhood. I can back out of my drive and right into hers. We are both 50. We have both been diagnosed with breast cancer in the last four months and have both had mastectomies. Now, Judi is dealing with chemical warfare. She has a lot to live for. Her oldest son, LJ, is 15 and is an excellent student. He is old enough and sensitive enough to her needs and hurts to be wonderful and comforting. Jay is 12, also a wonderful son. Jay plays football and the violin. He is a busy kid and gets busier as Judi goes through surgery and treatment, which is his way of dealing with the situation. Judi is taking control of everything she can, and that's a lot. That's why the hair was all cut off – it had started migrating from head to pillow, which was depressing for her to see. Having no hair is an adjustment, but she looks at its demise as evidence that the chemo is working. She regards the chemo as guerrilla warfare – a powerful gun shooting into a forest, hitting the good and bad alike. Once the enemy is gone, the good can regenerate and flourish again. We're looking forward to next spring when I can take the 'after' photo of Judi with new hair and new health. In the meantime life is good, with or without our hair, and we will live it to the fullest."

From the journal of Judy Von Bergen; diagnosed in 1997 at the age of 50; shopkeeper

Hats and Scarves

"I had quite a collection of hats, both for spring and winter. My collegues actually gave me a hat and scarf party! I really enjoyed wearing my spring hats. I would dress them up with scarves that matched my outfits. People at work looked forward to seeing what hat and scarf I would wear each day. Everyone from the chief executive to the security guards commented. It was great fun."
Val Long; diagnosed in 1999 at the age of 47; administrative assistant

"A friend of mine gave me a small fitted hat that was made of 100 per cent cotton and felt like T-shirt material. I did purchase a wig but found that it felt like a heavy, itchy swimming cap. I wore the hat around the house and to bed. Amazing how cold your head gets without any hair! When I went out, I mainly wore scarves. A friend made some for me, and I bought a few as well. My aunt also made some headcoverings that fit and felt perfect."
Gwen Loverink; diagnosed in 1994 at the age of 34; police dispatcher

"My single best purchase was a funky charcoal grey hat. It went with everything. I bought it at a hat and wig boutique owned by a cancer survivor. I credit Carol with my lack of self-consciousness with my 'no hair' look."
Rosamary Amiet; diagnosed in 2000 at the age of 48; programme manager

"Hats made it hard to hear, but I thought my wigs looked fake. Now, though, looking at pictures of me wearing my wigs, I think I looked pretty good. One advantage of the wigs: my hair was always perfect. But my hats were cool. I bought a dozen and wore a different one every day. I also bought big clip-on ear-rings and wore them every chance I got."
Betsy Goree; diagnosed in 1998 at the age of 40; magazine publisher/editor

"Two breast cancer survivors lent me their collection of hats for those long 'no hair' months. I accumulated a wardrobe of about three dozen hats – a veritable fashion show every day!"
Betty Harris; diagnosed in 1999 at the age of 64; housewife

"I wore hip children's hats. I also bought a wig, but did not care for that in the summer."
Candice Jaeger; diagnosed in 2000 at the age of 24; wife and mother

"I bought a wig, which I came to name 'the rat'. But it was just never comfortable – I decided that the distance from the top of my ears to the top of my head was too short – and it itched terribly. So I switched to scarves. A friend made me several scarves and also lent me tons of others. They were large – 34 inches square – so I could wrap them around my head twice."
Robin Smith; diagnosed in 2000 at the age of 53; microbiologist

"During the time I had no hair and while it was beginning to grow back, I wore turbans and scarves. It was summer and I was visiting my sister at the beach. Her seven-year-old grandson Scott was visiting also. Although he knew I was ill, he didn't know the details. He came over, sat next to me and asked why I was wearing a hat (actually, a turban). I told him it was hot and I just wanted to keep my hair out of the way. He said, 'Well, Aunt Carol, I think it looks really nice.' What a wonderful feeling came over me. I had often worried that the way I looked made the people around me uncomfortable."
Carol Englund; diagnosed in 1994 at the age of 58; retired administrative assistant

"I sometimes wore scarves, but most often wore a stretchy black velvet cap and then decorated it with colourful scarves to match my clothes or my mood. Once, when I was out to lunch with a friend, I wore a rather elaborately tied scarf on my head. The fabric matched my skirt and was rather chic. A woman at the table next to us complimented me on my 'hat' and wanted to know where she could buy one just like it."
Carrie Drake; diagnosed in 1998 at the age of 42; administrative assistant

"The best beach look? I always carried a scarf, so I wouldn't 'flip my wig' in an unexpected breeze. I did a great Jackie Onassis impression with big sunglasses and a scarf."
Sharon Carr; diagnosed in 1997 at the age of 42; hospice grief counsellor

"Some of us are confident or have a pretty enough shaped head to just go bald. But if you have to go through chemotherapy in the winter and you live anywhere the least bit chilly, you will want to cover your head. If you're lucky and really love your wig, then getting dressed will be easy. But if you're like me, your wig may not agree with you. Not only did my head itch and sweat, but the mirror reflected a strange and always crooked image. So scarves became my choice of cover-up. Once I learned how to tie them and adjust my wardrobe to match them, they actually became kind of fun."

Sallie Burdine; diagnosed in 1998 at the age of 44; author

"One day, I invited friends for dinner. They came dressed with bandanas on their heads, plus one for each of us. They even brought one for the dog! For Christmas and Chanukah, my partner's mum knitted the most outrageous hats, one for each day of the week. The entire family sat around the dinner table wearing some sort of head covering in pinks, reds, purples and greens. The men in the family looked absolutely smashing."

Carol Snyder; diagnosed in 1992 at the age of 47; special needs teacher

Wigs

"When my hair came out, I was a basket case. I thought I was prepared, but I was not. 'Hysterical' is how I would describe myself, but that was only for a few hours. Then I went home, put on my wig and no one really noticed that it *was* a wig. I got questions like 'Have you had a new haircut?' Not having hair is really no big deal. I'd just throw on a wig and go out."

Michele Marks; diagnosed in 1996 at the age of 33; CAD operator

"The very best thing about losing my hair during chemotherapy was the realisation that I could become a blonde, redhead, or brunette by purchasing wigs from a catalogue. This pleased me, since my natural brown colour was never to my liking. Also, with a wig, my 'hair' was always ready to go, so turning down an invitation was not an option. Getting out of the house was important."

Jean La Frombois; diagnosed in 1996 at the age of 57; part-time bookseller

"I most dreaded the whole experience of losing my hair and living bald in a world driven by cosmetic beauty. Little did I know what an experience it would become. I had gone shopping for a wig on my own once, and it was a terrible experience, so I decided I needed help. One Saturday, my daughters and I set out on our wig-finding adventure. We all tried on wigs and laughed at ourselves. It was hard to find a wig that resembled my own curly hair and looked nice, so my daughters convinced me to try a new style. It was a colour my hair was when I was younger, and much straighter than my hair has ever been. After scrunching it around on my still hairy scalp for a few minutes, I turned around, holding my breath and waiting for their reaction. The girls smiled approvingly and convinced me it was beautiful and made me look younger. Well, how could I resist looking younger?"

Ann Hurd; diagnosed in 1999 at the age of 57; dental surgery manager

"Buy your wig while you still have your own hair. When your hair starts to go, cut it, then shave your head. It makes you feel empowered."

Susan Rothstein; diagnosed in 1997 at the age of 49; travel agent

"Choose a wig that most flatters you, rather than one that closely replicates your current hairdo. The two may not be the same. Have an open mind, and don't be afraid to be daring. My wig was more glamorous than my own mop of hair, and my husband loved it."

Patricia Baker; diagnosed in 1993 at the age of 49; housewife

"My sister went with me to get a wig, and we laughed at the names of the wigs and those associations. Finally, I got two to have a choice."

Joanne Tutschek; diagnosed in 1998 at the age of 55; research communications director

"I went wig shopping with three of my friends and tried on all the hairdos that I never would have thought of wearing. I figured this was a great time to try out a new style. Before chemo, I had long, straight black hair. Instead of buying a wig like that, I got a platinum blonde wig for going out; a red one for work; and a pink, purple and blue one to wear when I got bored with the other two. When my friends and I went out, I would let them borrow whichever wigs I wasn't wearing myself. This way, I didn't feel as self-conscious. They were happy to help."

Asha Mevlana; diagnosed in 1999 at the age of 24; musician

"Getting a good wig can really boost your self-confidence. In the beginning, I couldn't imagine spending a lot of money on a hair-piece, especially if I was going to be ill and in the house a lot. Also, some people told me that wigs were itchy and uncomfortable. Well, mine wasn't. I felt pretty good after my first treatment and began to think that I shouldn't be stuck in the house because of the way I looked. I'm not a vain person, but I'd previously had so much hair that I had to cut it twice before it came out. So I bought a wig, and it made such a difference. Most people thought it was my natural hair, just straight now."

Donna Troiani; diagnosed in 2000 at the age of 42; part-time waitress, full-time mother

"Buy a more expensive wig, not a cheap one. It needs to look good for you to feel good. Also, have your wig fitted before you lose your hair. You will get a better fit for your head and will be able to match your natural colour."

Rhonda Sorrell; diagnosed in 1998 at the age of 43; special needs teacher

"Though hair loss will be temporary, even simple, matter-of-fact comments about its growing back offer no consolation. Give your-self time, and shop seriously for a wig. It will be 'you' for the next year. Take a friend with you, and you'll have a laugh and gain a valued opinion."

Mary Raffol; diagnosed in 1998 at the age of 44; teacher

"A friend who had gone through this a year before told me she had gone to a wig shop while her hair was the colour and style she liked. They made a wig to match exactly. I did as she suggested, and even though I didn't go through chemo, I felt prepared and in control. The wig has come in handy several times and is nice to have."

Carol Hattler; diagnosed in 1999 at the age of 65; retired nurse

"The wig problem was very stressful for me. I have a large head, so the majority of wigs didn't fit. A friend suggested a mail order cata-logue. This is a very nice and very private way to try on wigs!"

Sara Fallgren; diagnosed in 1978 at the age of 45; retired teacher

"How does a person who never really knew what to do with her

'original' hair prepare for the loss of hair that follows chemother-apy? First, I got my hairdresser to help me match a colour swatch to my current hair colour. Then, with her help I ordered a wig in a simple hairstyle that I felt I could keep in decent shape. The wig arrived, and I put it away until the day that I would need it. When I first noticed large quantities of my hair falling out, I called the local beautician's. They suggested that I come in within the hour so that they could shave off the hair that I had left. Off I went, in such a rush that I forgot my wig. But there was no turning back. The ladies got out the hair clippers and before I knew it I was completely bald. As quickly as the hair was brushed away, these same two angels placed a short, blonde, pixie-cut wig on my 64-year-old head. What fun! I had no time to whine or moan, as I had to get back to work. Well, the blonde wig was a huge success. It certainly didn't match my old hair colour, but it didn't make a bit of difference. Maybe it really is true that blondes have more fun!"
Florence Wade; diagnosed in 1999 at the age of 63; retired schoolteacher and property manager

"A little brown eyeshadow applied to the area around the hairline helps when wearing your wig."
Nan Comstock; diagnosed in 1988 at the age of 39; self-employed

"I wore a short wig in my usual hairstyle, so most people didn't know."
Becky Honeycutt; diagnosed in 1995 at the age of 53; nurse

"I loved my wigs! Everyone complimented me on my hairstyle, I never had to fuss about having a good hair day and being bald didn't bother me. I tried not to look in the mirror when the wig was removed, so it was not a concern."
Alyce Feinstein; diagnosed in 1993 at the age of 58; administrative assistant

"I had two wigs. One was a pageboy with a fringe, and the other was short, straight and layered. When my son was dressing up for Hallowe'en, he needed a wig, so I gave him the choice. He wore the pageboy and looked so good! The next day, I wore it myself and when I drove up to the school to pick up my younger son, both

boys' friends came up to me to tell me that they thought the wig looked better on Micah than on me!"
Jane Royal-Davidson; diagnosed in 1996 at the age of 47; teacher

"What got me through the difficult months of chemotherapy was making sure I always looked my best. I had purchased a great wig in a style very similar to my own hair. I went to each treatment wearing my beautiful wig, full make-up and a favourite trouser suit. The nurses constantly told me how healthy I looked, which was extremely uplifting. For me, looking my best was key to maintaining a positive outlook!"
Gail Rice; diagnosed in 1999 at the age of 48; teacher

"Here's a tip. Hold on to your wig when getting out of the back seat of a car or taxi, lest it catch on the clothing hook and you suddenly emerge bald."
Mindy Greenside; diagnosed in 2000 at the age of 48; midwife

"When wearing a wig, watch out for the oven. Pulling that pie out could melt your hair. Don't wear sweatshirts that go over your head, and forget changing rooms if you are trying on clothes that go over your head."
Ann Hurd; diagnosed in 1999 at the age of 57; dental surgery manager

There Is Something to Be Said for . . .

"I lost my hair on Mother's Day with 20 people coming to brunch. I really knew that the chemo was working – the hair loss proved it."
Debbie MacLean; diagnosed in 1991 at the age of 47; volunteer, hospital gift shop and hospice

"It was not so bad losing my hair. Oh, it was emotional at first. But then, look at how much time we women spend doing our hair. This was great. Toss on a wig or a hat, and that was that. And, oh, how my hair has grown back! It is great. Thick and curly. No more perms!"
Dee Pobjoy; diagnosed in 1999 at the age of 41; sales clerk

"There is something to be said for not having to shave our legs or pluck our eyebrows any more. I did have to learn how to draw eye-

brows, and if I had to pick, I would certainly pick 'plucking' over 'drawing'. But hey, I enjoyed the break."
Sallie Burdine; diagnosed in 1998 at the age of 44; author

"There were some good things about my hair falling out. First, my son learned he really wasn't adopted, since his hair growth pattern and mine match. Second, the hair on my legs grows less quickly now. Third, the hair under my arms never grew back, which is *not* a bad thing. Fourth, my son's wrestling team would rub my head for luck before a match; it felt good, and since I was comfortable, they were, too."
Jane Royal-Davidson; diagnosed in 1996 at the age of 47; teacher

"One week after my first chemo, my hair started falling out. I was so amazed that I could just pull it right out and it didn't even hurt. I didn't cry. I kept reminding myself that it was only temporary and that it would grow back. I said to myself, 'Think of all the money you'll save on shampoo! And you won't have to shave your legs or under your arms.' I laughed about that, and it made me feel better. I got a wig that was the exact same colour as my own hair. In fact, everyone thought the wig *was* my own hair! One day a friend called round. She said, 'You look so good! You haven't even lost your hair!' I took off the wig, and the look on her face was priceless. A few weeks after my last chemo, my hair started growing back. My head felt like a giant peach!"
Paula Porter; diagnosed in 2000 at the age of 47; telephone operator

"Rather than feel bad about my hair loss, I decided to sleep the extra hour in the morning. I did not need to blow-dry my hair or put mascara on, as I had no eyelashes – and I actually needed the extra sleep."
Jacki Anthony; diagnosed in 1998 at the age of 48; nurse

"After my treatments, our family took its annual July trip to the beach. Walking on the hot sand in my wig proved to be miserable. I traded my wig for a cute cap and continued with my holiday. When we went out for dinner, I would doll myself up with my wig and make-up, but I did not allow myself to become a prisoner of the situation. This was my holiday and I was determined to enjoy it."
Jean Joyce; diagnosed in 1999 at the age of 51; hairdresser, salon owner

"Funny thing about hair. They told me I would lose it, and I wanted to. That way, I wouldn't have to hear my husband say, 'When are you going to let your hair grow long?' But, guess what? It didn't fall out! It stopped growing and got a bit thin, but it stayed."
Pam Waddell; diagnosed in 1998 at the age of 38; writer, teacher's assistant

"When I was assured by the oncologist that my long blonde hair would fall out during chemo, I had it cut in a punk style and let my daughter dye it blue. When my scalp started to ache as the hair started to thin, I asked my son to buzz it with the clippers. We laughed together and cried together. When my hair had gone, friends gave me scarves that they had collected and I discovered that 22-inch dinner napkins were not only the perfect size, soft (100 per cent cotton) and washable, but they came in colourful prints that really lifted my spirits. Now that my hair is long enough to go without, I am making a quilt of all of the scarves."
Linda Jones Burns; diagnosed in 2000 at the age of 40; secondary school registrar

"I think about my friend who sent me a card saying that she would like a picture of me in my 'wig'. My thought is that I don't have 'a wig', I have 'hair'. I'm really attached to my hair. In fact, I need to use some more fabric conditioner on it."
Sandy Williams; diagnosed in 1999 at the age of 51; children's public librarian

"When my hair started falling out, I did not want my grandchildren to see me because I was afraid of what they would think. But they said they had friends who had lost their hair because of cancer and it was okay."
Wahnita Hawk; diagnosed in 1999 at the age of 56; nurse

"I had my head shaved just before Easter. My daughter Wendy brought Brittany, my six-year-old granddaughter, to see me. Brittany told her mum that I looked like an alien. I became her 'Alien Grandmother'. My other granddaughter, Sarah, who is four, didn't want to see me without my wig. I spent many hours with her just talking about my hair and wig, but she was adamant about it. One day, when we called in to visit, Brittany and Sarah were playing in the garage. As we left I pulled off my wig and said, 'Your Alien Grandmother says goodbye.' Sarah looked at me with her eyes and mouth open wide, unsure of what to do until she heard Brittany laughing. After that, it was all right to see me without my wig. Summer came, and I started to wear a hat, which she always wanted me to take off so she could feel my hair."

Nancy Ellis; diagnosed in 2000 at the age of 53; quality control technician

"You may lose your pubic hair with chemo. But it, too, grows back."

Monica May; diagnosed in 1997 at the age of 40; consultant

"I chose to be bald most of the time, rather than wearing a wig or scarf. When I went out, people would often ask me questions about my bald head. I gave my favourite response to a woman in a shop who asked me if I'd lost my hair. 'No,' I told her matter-of-factly. 'It's invisible.' She had nothing more to say."

Dorian Solot; diagnosed in 2000 at the age of 26

"During the time that I was wearing a wig because of chemotherapy, I had to tell a precious little eight-year-old that she had not got on to the gifted programme at school. It had been so important to her and I used every ploy, explanation and example I knew to make her understand that she was not a failure because of one test. But I couldn't get through to her. She was so sad, and the tears were still flowing. Finally, I said that she needed to count her blessings and be happy for the things she did have. When she still questioned herself, I pulled off my wig with a flourish and said, 'Look, you could be bald like me!' She collapsed laughing and promised not to say anything to the other pupils, because it might upset them. Today, that young lady is a very successful university student who left school with excellent grades. Although we had moved away by the time she left school, I received an invitation to her leaving party with a note thanking me for loving and encouraging her when she was a little girl."

Brenda Carr; diagnosed in 1988 at the age of 40; wife, mother, retired school counsellor

"Following my chemo treatments, I joined some other volunteer hairdressers in working with cancer victims. While giving classroom tips one day, I took a volunteer from the class and gave her a complete makeover. After marvelling at her appearance, she presented another wig on a foam head for me to style. I told her to put it on. She was a little embarrassed and did not want the class to see her switch wigs. I said, 'We will all turn our heads while you make the switch.' While everyone was turning their heads, I reached up and pulled my wig off, laying it on the table beside hers. You can image the surprise in the classroom when the women looked back up. They had only known me as 'Jean the Volunteer Beautician', not 'Jean the Cancer Survivor'. This was truly the icebreaker for my class. They immediately started opening up to me. One asked when I became comfortable taking my wig off in front of others. I told them, 'When I came to realise that there was so much more to life than a pretty head of hair.' "

Jean Joyce; diagnosed in 1999 at the age of 51; hairdresser, salon owner

Hair Again

"When my hair started coming back, random people on the street started commenting on how much they loved my haircut. They all thought I had such guts to cut it so short. Most of them said they had always wanted to try it but didn't have the courage to do it."

Asha Mevlana; diagnosed in 1999 at the age of 24; musician

"What a relief it was when my hair began to grow back. At first, I thought I'd go mad with the itching of my scalp. At times, wearing my wig was unbearable because of the itching. By Christmas, my hair resembled my son-in-law's number one cut. As the family was gathering for the holiday festivities I relaxed and took the itchy wig off. My seven-year-old granddaughter walked over and tried it on. She turned around, looking for all the world like Tina Turner, and, cocking her head on one side, announced, 'I don't think this is my style.' Today, my hair is thicker and less grey than it was before treatment. I will never complain about a 'bad hair day' again."

Ann Hurd; diagnosed in 1999 at the age of 57; dental surgery manager

"I didn't lose all my hair, but it was thin and so dry that it was three shades lighter. I made sure I got a good wash-and-wear haircut so I could stop blow-drying it, and it was back to its normal brown curly mop within a month of my last chemo treatment!"

Lynne Rutenberg; diagnosed in 1980 at the age of 35; retired teacher

"There was a time when my greatest fear was that my hair would never grow back. That was six years ago now and any complaint about a 'bad hair day' will never again be truly sincere."
Kathi Ward; diagnosed in 1994 at the age of 47; promotions executive

"When my treatment ended, my hair began to grow back. And you know what? I look great with short hair. I've always had long hair and never would have considered cutting it."
Linda Perkins; diagnosed in 1999 at the age of 35; project manager

"My beautician told me that when my hair started growing back, I shouldn't wear a wig or scarf when I was at home. She said that if you wear nothing on your head, your hair will grow back faster. She also said that massaging your head makes the hair grow back faster."
Paula Porter; diagnosed in 2000 at the age of 47; telephone operator

"I loved the first bit of fuzz when my hair started growing back. I felt like I was being given a chance to experience what I had gone through as a baby. It was incredible. My hair was so soft. If you haven't gone through this, it may sound a bit weird, but it was great. Like having been reborn and being allowed to experience it with all your senses. I loved it."
Val Long; diagnosed in 1999 at the age of 47; administrative assistant

"I liked my new curly hair so much, I have been having body waves ever since. My hair came back white, after having always been dark and dyed. My husband said, 'Well, at least we know what the real colour is!' "
Joanne Tutschek; diagnosed in 1998 at the age of 55; research communications director

"It's been a year and a half since I completed chemo for breast cancer. I had straight hair for 45 years, and now I have wonderful curly hair. It took nine months for my hair to grow back enough so that I didn't have to wear my wig."
A survivor; diagnosed in 1998 at the age of 45; dentist

"The second my hair had grown back enough to cover my head, I did away with the head coverings. It felt so good to feel the breeze

on my hair! It came back much thicker and curlier. Hardly takes me any time at all to style it now – just fluff and go!"
Gwen Loverink; diagnosed in 1994 at the age of 34; police dispatcher

"When my hair had gone, I didn't like wearing my wig and only did so when I was wearing 'grown-up' clothes. Other times I wore floppy-brimmed hats or went bare-headed. As soon as I had enough hair to cover my head – and look like a really chic haircut – I left the hats at home. My hair grew back evenly and, as it got longer, began to curl. The best part, though, was when friends and family who had watched me go through this would rub my new hair and curls. I knew that they were as thrilled to have that hair back as I was. And, of course, the hair only represented what we all wanted back and were thankful for – my health."
Faye Hardiman; diagnosed in 1998 at the age of 50; wife, mother, teacher

"When my hair started to fall out in clumps a couple of weeks after the first round of chemo, my husband used his beard-trimming kit to shave off the rest of it. I wore a cute wig when I went out or to work and a bandanna (often under a baseball cap) around the house and in the garden. The new hair was really curly, which was a wonderful surprise, and I stopped wearing the wig and bandanna for our first wedding anniversary weekend break!"
Beth Compton; diagnosed in 1995 at the age of 27; civil engineer

"I wore a little soft cotton stocking cap to sleep in. They can be purchased at a wig shop. That kept my head warm at night, and I felt 'protected' from the baldness. I didn't look at myself in the mirror much without my wig. I can't tell you how many people asked me where I got my hair cut. I actually grew so attached to my wig that it was hard for me to give it up. I was a redhead before the chemotherapy. Now my hair is a dark, dark brown. Before, my hair was limp and straight. Now I have waves and body. Sometimes I look in the mirror and wonder who I am!"
Sandy Williams; diagnosed in 1999 at the age of 51; children's public librarian

5 • Chemo and Everything Else

A Smorgasbord

Side effects. They're a pain. On one hand, you need the drugs to kill the cancer. On the other, the drugs kill some good stuff in the process. The result is tantamount to adding insult to the injury of a breast cancer diagnosis. What's the old saying, 'If the cancer doesn't get 'em, the cure will'? I certainly don't believe that. I wouldn't be bothering with this book if I did. No, I do believe in the cure. But I also believe that we need to deal with those unfortunate side effects.

The last chapter talked about hair loss. This chapter deals with the rest – a broad group that includes stomach upset, fatigue and a couple of other little things that are totally annoying. For starters, there's *nothing* worse than taking medication and experiencing side effects that may be perfectly normal but that no one has warned you about! Lauren Nichols, a writer who was diagnosed in 2000 at the age of 53, had that experience during chemotherapy.

"The anti-nausea drugs I was given before my first treatment not only made me sick but wired me so badly that deep inside myself, I was bouncing off the walls. The awful thing is, I didn't realise I wasn't supposed to feel that way, so I did the 'stiff upper lip' thing and said nothing until my follow-up check-up. That's when the nurse told me that some people have what amounts to an allergic reaction to certain drugs. They put me on something else and it worked well."

In this instance, as in others mentioned later in this chapter, a simple switch of anti-nausea medication solved the problem. Unfortunately, the chemo itself can't be switched. There just aren't enough drugs with the same ability to cure without those side effects. And not all women experience them. Every woman's body is different, which is possibly why medical advances in treating female ailments have been slow in coming — but that's another story entirely. Suffice it to say here that one woman's body may experience a side effect that another woman's never will. That said, there's no harm keeping *UPLIFT* nearby just in case — because while the medical community searches for antidotes to side effects, survivors have their own ideas. Call them folk remedies, but, hey, if they work . . .

The most common side effects of chemo are well known — namely, hair loss and nausea. But there is another one that takes people by surprise. Michele Marks, who was diagnosed in 1996 at the age of 33, broached it first. "When I went through chemo, no one told me I might have trouble remembering things or get distracted easily. It's chemo-brain, and it explains a lot. I found half-finished notes and longer things that I started but didn't finish, and I couldn't think of words or remember things. For a while I thought I was going mad. It was chemo-brain. But nobody told me then."

Betsy Goree, who was diagnosed in 1998 at the age of 40, elaborated: "Simply put, chemo-brain is the way your brain reacts to the chemo drugs. Chemo-brain makes you forgetful. You might feel as if you are coming down with Alzheimer's (don't worry, it's only cancer) because you can't recall a song title or your next-door neighbour's name. You may have a hard time finishing a sentence, or remembering your dog's name or what you went to the shop for. This is annoying. It is especially bad when your loved ones give you the look that says 'chemo-brain' (so try not to do that, everyone). This look used to upset me because I would realise that I had forgotten something (again). I don't forget nearly as much any more, but if I do, I just say to myself, 'Chemo-brain is real. You have it because you had cancer and you went to great lengths to kill the cancer. How important is that 1940s film star's name anyway?' Sometimes when I am alone in my car, I say this out loud, then look at myself – and all my hair – in the rear view mirror and say, 'You had cancer?' "

Betsy skips a line, then adds, "The good thing about chemo-brain is that it goes away."

This sentiment is shared by Linda Perkins, who was diagnosed in 1999 at the age of 35. "The gradual end of chemo-brain and the return of my short-term memory reminds me daily of my good fortune and the light at the end of the tunnel."

Which just goes to show that the glass can be half full even when you can't remember putting any water in it at all!

Which has absolutely nothing to do with smoking pot.

Though I've heard that that does help curb nausea . . .

Keeping It Down

"Always eat before going to chemo. Nausea is more acute with an empty stomach and it is often difficult to eat after the treatment. For that reason, eat whatever you want whenever you can. Nutrition is important, but your regular diet may not be palatable. Comfort foods that line the stomach make a difference – rice, potatoes, pasta."
Patricia Baker; diagnosed in 1993 at the age of 49; housewife

"What works best for me in the nausea department is keeping my stomach full just before treatment and for two days after it. I also drink plenty of water before treatment. I eat a light breakfast, and if I have to wait for a long time, I bring dry biscuits to munch on before I go in. Carbohydrates seem to do it for me at this time. Lots of bread is not good for the waistline, but . . ."
Donna Troiani; diagnosed in 2000 at the age of 42; part-time waitress, full-time mother

"The Christmas after my surgery, my Christmas card to my former college room-mate crossed paths with hers to me. Both contained the same message – that we had had mastectomies that year. Her advice to me was to keep my stomach full. I ate muffins by the dozen, and it helped."
Jane Vaughan; diagnosed in 1991 at the age of 53; writer

"A friend told me to drink two litres of tonic water over two days following the chemo infusion. The quinine in the water was like a

miracle. No more leg and foot pains. I mixed it with orange juice and sipped it. What a difference!"
Phyllis Jezequel; diagnosed in 1999 at the age of 66; missionary

"What helped me get through my diagnosis, five operations and nine months of treatment for breast cancer, at the age of 35? The three Gs – God and plenty of faith, Ginger (crystallised) to help the nausea from the treatment and Garlic. And, of course, Jewish penicillin (chicken soup) on a regular basis."
Linda Perkins; diagnosed in 1999 at the age of 35; project manager

"My absolute standby for food when I felt sick was cream crackers. I also always kept packets of instant oatmeal on hand to pop into the microwave. Oatmeal is bland and filling, and the packets were great to take to work. Lollies were good, too. I was always thirsty!"
Deborah Lambert; diagnosed in 2000 at the age of 47; medical secretary

"My friend Tammy was told to drink lots of water. This gives you beautiful skin, which is important, since people are more apt to notice your skin when you have no hair."
Nanette Carter; friend of Tammy Blackwell

"I had read in a book that eating an ice lolly during treatment helps with the gum soreness that I had after my first treatment. So I went to the second treatment lollies in hand, but they melted. I had a very cold ginger ale and resorted to swishing that round my mouth, and the truth is it did help."
Donna Troiani; diagnosed in 2000 at the age of 42; part-time waitress, full-time mother

"During chemotherapy, suck on ice cubes for a few minutes while the solution is first entering your veins. This actually works to eliminate mouth sores."
Cheryl Cavallo; diagnosed in 1997 at the age of 35; housewife

"Ice lollies immediately before my chemotherapy froze the cells in my mouth and prevented me from getting mouth sores. The treatment also resulted in vaginal dryness, which can be very painful for a young woman. Thank goodness for vaginal lubricants!"
Linda Perkins; diagnosed in 1999 at 35; project manager

"Aromatherapy helps with nausea, especially Vicks VapoRub under the nose and on the throat."
Elaine Raco Chase; friend of many survivors

"For chemo, I would always bring an extra-large iced coffee and sip away. It is important to have lots of liquids. If possible, bring someone with a great sense of humour – a good friend or family member to share the time with."
Rayna Ragonetti; diagnosed in 1993 at the age of 52; executive

"Chicken soup was the only meal I ever ate after chemo treatment and it never made me sick."
Penny Trosterman; diagnosed in 1996 at the age of 45; English teacher

"My favourite food during chemo was Mexican food. It had spice in it that I could taste through the 'metal' mouth that chemo causes. I also ate a lot of ice cream. It felt good to have something cold in my mouth, especially when I had mouth sores. Overall, though, I pretty much ate whatever I could whenever I could. On the good days, I tried to make up for the bad days, so my goal was to get as many calories into my system as I could."
Gwen Loverink; diagnosed in 1994 at the age of 34; police dispatcher

"Eat cold, raw foods during chemo treatment. Carrot sticks, celery, ham sandwiches – anything that doesn't have a strong odour. Hot foods with a strong smell can make nausea seem worse. Also, breathe through your mouth if odours begin to bother you. The clinic where I had chemo treatments always had coffee going in the lobby. I couldn't stand the smell of it after two treatments. I started breathing through my mouth so the smell wouldn't bother me. When I had a funny taste in my mouth, I sucked peppermints."
Jennifer Wersal; diagnosed in 2000 at the age of 30; marketing

"During chemo, stick to a light diet. After my first treatment, I ate spaghetti, and that did not work. Drink lots of juice and ice-cold tea."
Mary Ann Lee; diagnosed in 1988 at the age of 46; tax collector

"For a while, nothing at all tasted good and I could only stomach ice lollies. Then there was a period when grilled cheese sandwiches and jelly were all I could eat. Then frozen macaroni and cheese tasted good. It was months before I could enjoy a good steak, a nice salad and a glass of red wine – but when I did, I savoured every mouthful."

Carrie Drake; diagnosed in 1998 at the age of 42; administrative assistant

"Eating tofu during my recovery gave me a wonderful boost. I could actually feel myself healing after a tofu milkshake. It eased the tissues. Most people douse tofu with soy sauce and fry it until it tastes horrible. I invented putting a slice of tofu (as thick as a slice of bread) in a blender along with a half cup of pineapple, a banana, and a glass of milk or juice. Beat it, and it comes out thick and creamy and delicious. That was usually my breakfast or lunch."

Lorraine J. Pakkala-Lintala; diagnosed in 1992 at the age of 62; editor, author

"A neighbour had breast cancer. While going through chemo, she was able to keep organic oatmeal down, cooked on the thin side. It's soothing to the stomach and strengthens the body – vital when it's being zapped by chemo and radiotherapy. I also noticed that she gained some weight during the break between her chemo and radiation treatments. I thought she looked great and told her so. She said she'd been purposely eating more in order to gain weight, so when she had the inevitable weight loss, she'd be pretty much at her normal weight. Very clever. She never had an emaciated look – never looked like a patient at all!"

Nancy Summersong; friend of a survivor

"I was surprised that my appetite was so good. I expected to lose weight during chemotherapy. In fact, I was sort of counting on it. Big disappointment. The first week after I recovered from chemo, I wanted to eat everything in sight, and usually did. The first food I craved was a McDonald's fish fillet sandwich. Talk about weird. After my fourth and fifth chemos, I wanted potato salad, which was even weirder, since I had never eaten it before. The foods I wanted and could eat seemed to change during the course of the chemo. My rule of thumb was that if my brain and my stomach agreed on something, I would eat it."

Val Long; diagnosed in 1999 at the age of 47; administrative assistant

"The biggest surprise: despite heavy-duty chemo, surgery and radiotherapy, nothing was as bad as I thought it might be. I never even threw up once! The new drugs are wonderful and ginger tea helped my stomach before it even thought of acting up."
Sharon Carr; diagnosed in 1997 at the age of 42; hospice grief counsellor

"Being one of the lucky people who did not feel sick with chemotherapy, I was determined to keep up my strength with lots of protein and dairy products. When the hospital dietitian said to me during one of my chemo treatments, 'Jean, I really don't think you need all those cheeseburgers and shakes – you weigh a little too much,' I knew I wasn't wasting away!"
Jean La Frombois; diagnosed in 1996 at the age of 57; part-time bookseller

"After my first chemo, I went home and threw up for three days. A friend had come to be with me after the chemo, and we joked that this was the way to get rid of that extra stone I'd been trying desperately to lose. For the remaining chemo sessions, I asked for more anti-nausea medication and didn't throw up again."
Patti R. Martinez; diagnosed in 1999 at the age of 54; estate agent

"What helped most for the nausea was walking, breathing cool clean air, making myself move. I'd have a treatment and my husband would come home and say, 'Hey! You need a walk.' And he would pull me out of the door, but I did feel much better."
Pam Waddell; diagnosed in 1998 at the age of 38; writer, teacher's assistant

Magic Bullets

"The only foods that tasted good to me when I was on chemo were spaghetti and pudding. I ate them every day."
Paula Porter; diagnosed in 2000 at the age of 47; telephone operator

"Tuna fish and chicken noodle soup were great feel-better foods for me after a round of chemo. Chocolate chip cookies were a great soother, too."
Kathy Rabassa; diagnosed in 1999 at the age of 34; administrative assistant

"Having cream crackers to chew on and a bottle of flat Coke under my desk at work kept me going during chemo."
Alysa Cummings; diagnosed in 1998 at the age of 45; educational trainer

"A glass of chocolate milk helped me during chemo."
Pam Waddell; diagnosed in 1998 at the age of 38; writer, teacher's assistant

"I craved cottage cheese. It made me feel good to eat it, and eat it I did. It did not make me feel sick when I was having chemo. I ate it by the gallon."
Judy Komitee; diagnosed in 1998 at the age of 52; secretary

"I swear by my Chinese tea and believe it is a huge contributing factor to my not having nausea at all during chemo."
Sandy Rodgers; diagnosed in 1999 at the age of 44; mother, nurse, Reiki master

"For me, it helped to eat a big lunch before chemo and to drink pop or my favourite grapefruit juice during chemo."
A survivor; diagnosed in 1998 at the age of 45; dentist

"My favourite food was a doughnut. I'm not sure why, but it helped my stomach. Cream crackers helped if I felt sick."
Mary Ann Budnick; diagnosed in 1991 at the age of 44; school bus driver

"Sucking on boiled sweets during treatment helped me minimise the nausea of chemotherapy."
Nan Comstock; diagnosed in 1988 at the age of 39; self-employed

"My favourite food was a boiled potato. It helped with the nausea."
Frances Gallello; diagnosed in 2000 at the age of 51; mental health assistant

"I ate lots of apple sauce, and actually gained over half a stone during my last three months of chemo!"
Rosamary Amiet; diagnosed in 2000 at the age of 48; programme manager

"When my cousin was going through chemo, she only wanted thick chocolate milkshakes."
Donna Krol; cousin of survivor

"I had a cup of coffee and a doughnut with my treatments, and I drank lots and lots of water."
Susan Schultz; diagnosed in 1990 at the age of 41; special needs teacher's assistant

"Lots of ginger, ginger tea, biscuits and nuts all help with nausea."
Mindy Greenside; diagnosed in 2000 at the age of 48; midwife

"My favourite things to eat and drink during treatment were ginger ale and biscuits. I ate yogurt every day to combat mouth sores and diarrhoea, neither of which I ever got."
Deborah J. P. Schur; diagnosed in 1994 at the age of 43; sales rep

"With chemo, I gained so much water weight – once it was nearly a stone. So I ate watermelon, which is a natural diuretic, and I lost all the weight in two days."
Judith Ormond; diagnosed in 1996 at the age of 49; symphony musician – piccolo

Staying Upbeat

"Think positive. Chemo is something they do *for you*, not *to* you. Chemo is a weapon in a war. You are taking control by submitting to chemo. You are now the aggressor. Each treatment is a bombardment of the enemy. When you really feel lousy, then you know the weapon is doing a good job attacking that enemy."
Patricia Baker; diagnosed in 1993 at the age of 49; housewife

"I used Pac Man as imagery to eat up any errant cancer cells during chemo. When I walked, which I did almost every day (I think that really helped with fatigue too), I would picture those little guys gobbling up all those bad cells growing in and around lots of my organs and bones."
Robin Smith; diagnosed in 2000 at the age of 53; microbiologist

"My friends came to all my treatments and helped pass the time. We ordered food and watched films, which made everything much more tolerable."
Asha Mevlana; diagnosed in 1999 at the age of 24; musician

"If you have to spend a prolonged stretch in the hospital, bring music with you. Music can be a tonic or a tranquilliser. It's an effective, healthy mood enhancer with no bad side effects."
Barbara Keiler; sister and daughter of a survivor

"I felt a 100 years old after eight rounds of chemo. No one could explain why. Finally, a doctor at another medical centre said that about a quarter of his patients felt like this for no known reason after the completion of chemo."
Monica May; diagnosed in 1997 at the age of 40; consultant

"I always applied skincare products and make-up daily, so I never looked ill. Friends would always comment on how good I looked, and before long I started feeling that way."
Cheryl Cavallo; diagnosed in 1997 at the age of 35; housewife

"Make-up, make-up, make-up! Nothing helps to restore your sense of femininity more than a face that looks better than people expect it to. Eyeliner disguises the loss of your eyelashes, and a fringe on a wig hides disappearing eyebrows. Do anything not to feel like a patient. Always get dressed and groomed in the morning, even on the bad days. With the greatly improved anti-nausea medication, life can go on. I never missed a party. Even if I couldn't eat the hors d'oeuvres, the festive company took me out of myself, and my family and I were better for it."
Patricia Baker; diagnosed in 1993 at the age of 49; housewife

"I put on make-up every day. A good eyeliner pencil works wonders when your eyelashes have gone. Draw on eyebrows, then use a brow brush to make them look real. Don't do what I did several times – accidentally rub one of your brows off! I still laugh about that. Remember to smile every day. It feels good!"
Sherry Ann Wells; diagnosed in 1997 at the age of 45; housewife

"My first round of chemo, the nausea drug worked okay *if* I could take it and keep it down. I took an immediate dislike to the look of the pill, and I've never been very good at taking pills anyway. I'm a gagger, and just the thought of taking something four times a day would get me started. The second round of chemo, they gave me a

new drug. This was like a miracle. First, I liked the way it looked. Second, I only had to take it twice a day."
Val Long; diagnosed in 1999 at the age of 47; administrative assistant

"I did not tolerate chemo well. When the drugs make you sick and nothing helps, you just want to end the suffering. Then I looked at the faces of my two Corgi dogs, and I knew I could not leave my husband and them. I decided that I could beat this. Sure enough, we found an anti-nausea drug that helped."
Kathy Rabassa; diagnosed in 1999 at the age of 34; administrative assistant

"For hot flushes brought on by chemo, invest in a powerful air conditioner and wear cotton clothing."
Penny Trosterman; diagnosed in 1996 at the age of 45; English teacher

"I gained weight during treatment; now I've lost it again. What a great feeling!"
Linda Perkins; diagnosed in 1999 at 35; project manager

"Camisole tops made of a nice silk were my favourites during treatment. I bought several loose jackets and blouses like jackets, and wore them over the tops or a dress."
Carol Hattler; diagnosed in 1999 at the age of 65; retired nurse

"It's important to have really comfortable pyjamas. I did a lot of lounging around at home, and almost never took off my purple flannel pyjamas."
Asha Mevlana; diagnosed in 1999 at the age of 24; musician

"For chemo sessions, I wore T-shirts from exciting events or trips. They were a sort of talisman."
Judith Ormond; diagnosed in 1996 at the age of 49; symphony musician – piccolo

"I covered my baldness with a funny hat. For each day of treatment I wore a different cartoon T-shirt. My favourite was Goofy! At the last treatment, I gave cartoon T-shirts to all the staff."
Carol Snyder; diagnosed in 1992 at the age of 47; special needs teacher

"On the days of chemotherapy, I would finish my treatment, have lunch with family, friends or colleagues, and then go home and have a quick nap. That weekend, we always planned a fun trip or event. This way the attention was taken away from me and placed on a fun family outing. Not only did it entertain the kids, but I also enjoyed these outings. Also, on the night before most of my chemotherapy treatments, I would have a full-body massage to help relax and renew me. Later, I learned that Reiki is very helpful before treatments. I have since become a Reiki practitioner and help other women before they have their chemotherapy."

Deborah J. P. Schur; diagnosed in 1994 at the age of 43; sales rep

"During chemo, you'd be better off not using your fingers to apply make-up. Instead, use a sponge or disposable applicator. Discard make-up that you used before chemotherapy, as it may contain bacteria that your body can no longer ward off because of the drop in white blood count. When defences are down, it is also a good idea to open a new mascara every three months."

Jean Joyce; diagnosed in 1999 at the age of 51; hairdresser, salon owner

"Can someone tell me how to lose weight while I'm taking Tamoxifen? I have to take it for two more years. But then, needing to lose weight isn't so bad. I'm alive and plan to stay that way for many years to come."

Penny Trosterman; diagnosed in 1996 at the age of 45; English teacher

6 • Taking the Reins

Regaining Control

Loss of control is a major issue for those with breast cancer. It starts early on, when a problem is first suspected, and suddenly we're taken over by fear, not to mention mammography machines, localisation needles, hospital release forms and biopsies. Then a positive diagnosis comes and we're *really* hit for six. We're swamped by new information, confused by choices, intimidated by sterile rooms. We worry enough to lose sleep; we're hurting from operations, weak from anaesthetics, and stressed about family demands; and we are not looking forward to the treatment ahead. There's this big . . . big 'C' looming over us, crushing us under its weight, threatening to dominate our daily lives for the foreseeable future.

But stop. Take a breath. Tell yourself that you *have* to be positive, because you're the one in the driving seat here. Oh, you may have to work at it a little, and the change may not take place overnight. Being positive can take practice. More than anyone else, though, *you* can make it happen.

"You need to set the tone," wrote Anne Jacobs, managing partner of an estate agency. "I found that being upbeat, coming to therapy with a smile on my face, being interested and communicating that interest to the people around me had an uplifting effect on everyone. I remember feeling down one day in the lift on the way to therapy. As the doors opened I forced a big smile. My whole body responded and I bounced into the waiting area. I felt in control."

Jane Royal-Davidson, a teacher, came at it a different way. "I was more frightened by the chemo than the cancer, but I had been told by my friend, a doctor, that I was the driver of the train. I had complete control. So I let only those people who were supportive on the train and left those who were uncomfortable off. I could control cancer, or it would control me. I chose to have control."

Cathleen D'Antonio, who learned she had breast cancer in 1994, was 28 at the time. "Being diagnosed was a huge shock," she wrote. "But instead of dwelling on the 'Why me?' factor, I saved my energies for tackling the disease. One of the things that has helped me over the years is accepting that there are going to be some dark days. The light at the end of the tunnel comes from knowing that I have nephews, nieces, parents and other family members who are always there to give me a laugh, a shoulder to cry on or an ear to listen. I was just going through a rough break-up when I was diagnosed. Even in my sadness, I learned that I was a great person, that I could enjoy being myself."

Someone else learned it, too. In his own contribution to UPLIFT, Cathleen's husband, Mark D'Antonio, writes, "I fell in love with my wife one year after her diagnosis . . ."

Which is proof that having a positive attitude does more than beat cancer.

So, there's determination, imagery and love. There are also some more concrete things that we can do. Cornelia Doherty, a 16-year survivor, recalls, "I needed to have some control in a situation over which I had no control. So I decided that I would drive myself to every one of my chemo treatments and to every day of radiotherapy. Many, many people wanted to help me, but it gave me great strength to do it myself."

Florence Wade, who was diagnosed in 1999, regained control by keeping busy with things that made her happy. "I read two or three novels each week, kept a diary now and then, and put together a grandmother's memory book, which I had copied and bound for each of my four grandchildren."

Helaine Hemingway, who was diagnosed at the age of 41, tells how she regained control. "Long-term goals were helpful. I continued to teach and work on my post-graduate qualification."

What did I do to regain control? I've been thinking about that a lot. I mean, I told you that I got my own tattoo, which satisfied my need to thumb my nose at those other little blue ones. And the sports car. . . . Oh. I didn't mention that? Well, I needed a new car anyway, and the boys had grown up and had cars of their own, and I'd always wanted a sports car but had never thought they were safe enough. Then it struck me that *I'd had cancer*. I could do what I wanted to do. So I bought the car, and all these years later I still own it, despite the objections of our oldest son, who never tires of arguing that it would be much happier in the South (with his wife and him), than in the cold and stormy Northeast.

Sorry, Eric. That baby's mine. For me, that sports car is a symbol of health, strength and freedom from fear. It also represents the broader tactic that helped me regain control when cancer tried to rob me of it – defiance.

Is "defiance" too strong a word? Try 'boldness'. Boldness enabled me to say, 'Yes, I want a sports car!' It also allowed me to do a lot of smaller things that really helped – like finding a dressmaker with whom I was comfortable enough to be able to say, "I've had breast cancer and reconstruction, so I'd like you to alter the darts on the front of this dress to fit my new breasts," and looking a pushy saleswoman in the eye and saying, "Yes, I know that I'm young enough to wear that barely-there swimming costume you're holding, but I've had breast cancer and reconstruction, and I'm not quite comfortable with that particular upper half." That shut *her up* fast! Actually, my speaking up worked like a charm in both cases; both women were understanding and solicitous. Quite frankly, I cannot imagine another woman being anything but understanding and solicitous when she's told something like that.

In an attempt to remember other things that I'd done during those months that helped with the issue of control, I went through my stash of old calendars and pulled out the ones that had hung on the kitchen wall during the years of my operations and treatment. Well, we went to dinner with friends, and we went to family events. We went on weekend trips for my husband's legal firm. I gave some local speeches, plus one further afield. I went to cousins' lunches, to the dentist's, to the optician's. I had my car serviced. I went with son No.1 when he had his wisdom teeth out, and son No. 2 when he needed clothes, and son No. 3 to have some Thai food. I had my hair cut. I had my hair highlighted. I had my nails done – actually had them done every week during that whole time and still do – and I make no apologies for the indulgence. With my hands on a keyboard all day long, I see my fingernails more than any other part of my body!

So, there were no clues to coping with cancer on my calendars. They were filled with the normal day-to-day workings of my life, which were not particularly different from the years before or since.

Of course . . . you guessed it. The remarkable thing was the *absence* of cancer on those pages. I actually had to struggle to reconstruct that journey – the dates of biopsies, operation planning sessions, the start of radiotherapy. The only note on my calendar that marked my mastectomy was a large squiggle over the day. Two days after that, the twins turned 21. They were away at college. I remember sending them gift baskets of cheese, biscuits and beer. Not that beer took precedence over cancer, but my sons' 21st birthday certainly did!

Studying those calendars, I realised that my method of coping with cancer had been to continue with the rest of my life. Oh, yeah, I did work out that "2 p.m. with Dr Y" meant an appointment with my plastic surgeon for saline injections. But notes like that weren't prominent. They were entered on those calendars in the same small print that I used to mark when the pest control man was due for his quarterly visit. "Everything looks good, Mrs D. A few mice in the garage, comin' in from the cold, but we can live with that."

I certainly can.

Feeling Good about Ourselves

"What made me feel feminine again? Aromatherapy – scented candles and a nice hot bath sprinkled with scented bathsalts and oils. Also, sexy lingerie worn under lace or velvet tops."
Carrie Drake; diagnosed in 1998 at the age of 42; administrative assistant

"The best thing that I do for myself right now is to use a foamy body wash in the shower so that those bubbles of foam cover my body. I love that feeling."
Susan Smith; diagnosed in 2000 at the age of 53; medical library technician

"After my surgery, I learned to enjoy the luxury of a long hot shower. I had always been in too much of a hurry to allow myself to stay in the shower for 10 to 15 minutes!"
Wanda Null; diagnosed in 1986 at the age of 41; librarian

"Never underestimate the value of a good shopping spree – by catalogue from home, if necessary."
Susan Rothstein; diagnosed in 1997 at the age of 49; travel agent

"One of my fondest memories was strutting into a lingerie shop to find the sexiest black lace bra they had . . . the more expensive the better."
Kathi Ward; diagnosed in 1994 at the age of 47; promotions executive

"The main thing we all need to remember is to rest and eat. I was always one to go, go, go, and now this is the time to relax and enjoy life. That is how I feel to this day. Life is precious."
Candice Jaeger; diagnosed in 2000 at the age of 24; wife and mother

"Get a massage or a pedicure or both. I did, and it really gave me something to look forward to. If you've just had surgery, you might consider reflexology. It is a massage of the feet that lasts an hour and relaxes the entire body. You will be very comfortable and not have to worry about the operation site."
Rhonda Sorrell; diagnosed in 1998 at the age of 43; special needs teacher

"I bought several beautiful nightdresses, a fabulous wig, great hats and new make-up. I always wore the wig and I always dressed impeccably, no matter how awful I felt. It was important to me that no one thought of me as ill."
Cornelia Doherty; diagnosed in 1985 at the age of 45; mother, widow, speaker

"My advice? Do not sit back feeling sorry for yourself. Take one day at a time, and do all you can to live as normally as possible. For me, that meant looking my best every day. I wore a nice wig and made sure that my make-up was on the minute I was out of the shower. I felt very special when I did this."
Carol Downer; diagnosed in 1997 at the age of 48; legal secretary

"When I left the hospital, I was determined to look my best – and I succeeded, although I crawled into bed when I got home and slept for four hours! I knew that if I felt good about my appearance, it would speed my recovery. When I became tired or my incision hurt, I learned to take care of myself by lessening physical activity until I felt stronger. The long-term effect is that my house isn't as clean as it used to be, and there is definitely more clutter, but I am comfortable with that."
Wanda Null; diagnosed in 1986 at the age of 41; librarian

"Hire a housekeeper once a week. Save your strength for your family."
Rhonda Sorrell; diagnosed in 1998 at the age of 43; special needs teacher

"The most practical thing that I've done for myself since last year is to have my house cleaned professionally every two weeks. The two hours that it takes two women to do an excellent job saves me the stress of wanting a clean house while juggling the need to have fun and still working full time."
Christine Foutris; diagnosed in 1999 at the age of 49; teacher

"The advice that I would give to a friend? Spring clean. Spring clean your inner and outer house, meaning your mind and your body, to make room for new positive thoughts and actions."
Carol Pasternak; diagnosed in 1986 at the age of 47; artist

"Acupuncture helped me overcome fatigue. I also tried heal-touch therapy and had massages. It's good to feel cared for."
Judith Ormond; diagnosed in 1996 at the age of 49; symphony musician – piccolo

"Walking and meditation helped me a lot. There was a great group meditation in my ten-week mind–body class, and they gave us individual tapes for meditation, since it was difficult to get my mind to concentrate enough to do it myself. Also, to help feel in control, I attended discussion groups, swimming therapy and yoga for cancer patients, plus a wonderful support group that I still attend at the cancer centre."
Joanne Tutschek; diagnosed in 1998 at the age of 55; research communications director

"I read a book that opened my eyes to the connection between diet and cancer. I changed my diet completely after reading it. I used to be a junk food junkie, eating whatever I wanted whenever I wanted. Now, I am almost a total vegetarian – eating only organic turkey occasionally, and organic eggs and raw goat's milk cheese. I don't eat out any more and I cook everything from scratch. In spite of the cancer, I feel better than I have in the last ten years. I wouldn't change this for anything."
A survivor; diagnosed in 2000 at the age of 43; teacher

"During my hospital stay, I was quite a health nut. I took vitamins E and C daily, ate garlic regularly, and believed that tofu was the food of the gods. I watched other people in the ward have crisps and Coke for breakfast. They were always awake in the night complaining of indigestion and restlessness."
Lorraine J. Pakkala-Lintala; diagnosed in 1992 at the age of 62; editor, author

"I had a need to control something, and walking helped. That was 'my' time. An hour with earphones and music helped reduce anxiety. I focused on eating more healthily. That was something else I could control. I also made a decision to smile every time I looked in a mirror, and I soon found that I smiled a lot and that the reflection looking back at me no longer seemed so frightened."
Pauline Hughes; diagnosed in 1997 at the age of 61; retired nurse

"I felt most in control when I was pulling up weeds in my front garden. This 'therapy' was mindless but productive work that allowed for a lot of daydreaming. I likened pulling up weeds to killing cancer cells. I still love to weed."
Beth Compton; diagnosed in 1995 at the age of 27; civil engineer

"These days the sun seems brighter and the sky bluer. I continue to plan ahead, as it helps me to have something to look forward to. Hiking and driving in the mountains is the best medicine around!"
Judy Peterson; diagnosed in 2000 at the age of 58; nurse

"Being a couch potato is okay, too! You don't have to do anything – fighting cancer is enough."
Linda Perkins; diagnosed in 1999 at the age of 35; project manager

"I continued to work, write letters and shop even though I did feel tired sometimes. Good food, good friends and a loving family made it all worthwhile."

Marge Fuller; diagnosed in 1994 at the age of 63; education authority official, retired

"I think the best thing you can do to regain control is to live your life as you did before. Go to church, go to weddings, visit your family, play with your children or grandchildren, take drives to the mountains. Read or walk. My husband would take me for ice cream frequently during chemotherapy. I know one woman whose husband took her dancing every week when she was undergoing cobalt treatments many, many years ago."

Faye Hardiman; diagnosed in 1998 at the age of 50; wife, mother, teacher

"After having a mastectomy, I was devastated to learn that I would have to go through months of chemotherapy. So I found a project to do. My wardrobe shelves were lined with boxes of my two daughters' memorabilia, from their first drawings to their college scrapbooks. My husband, Fred, joined in to write special messages of our memories of different events. These were albums of love and hope for me, my own special therapy, and it worked! I realised that there were still so many memories to make with my family, and it made me strong."

Carol Merrill; diagnosed in 1996 at the age of 48; housewife

"What kept my friends and relatives so supportive was their seeing me out doing things and not feeling down. I was determined not to put my life on hold. Four days after my first chemo treatment, my husband and I went camping. Three days after coming home from hospital after my mastectomy, I went out to dinner. People were surprised to see me out, but I felt good. A positive attitude helps the healing process."

Diane Zellar; diagnosed in 2000 at the age of 51; housewife

Reading, Writing and Reasoning

"What helped pass time in lieu of worrying? For me it was reading. I read tons of books. It was a great escape."

Gwen Loverink; diagnosed in 1994 at the age of 34; police dispatcher

"I often felt saddest at bedtime, when my mind would fill with fear. I found it helped to read before bed each night to help replace the terror with other thoughts and images. My favourite reads turned out to be what I called 'comfort food books' – novels I'd read before and loved. Although usually I rarely reread books, during this time it felt too overwhelming to focus on new books, particularly since so many plots involve tragedy and death, either of which would have made me feel worse. Returning to the pages of old friends was comforting and safe, often evoking warm memories of the first time I'd enjoyed the book. A five-minute reading dose each night brought a noticeable decrease in the number of nightly tears on my pillow and panic-filled cancer dreams."
Dorian Solot; diagnosed in 2000 at the age of 26

"Having a creative project that doesn't give you time to feel sorry for yourself after surgery is a wonderful help. I write a mystery series about an absent-minded sleuth, and the deadline for the fifth book in the series was six months after the mastectomy. So I immersed myself in my writing."
Elizabeth Daniels Squire; diagnosed in 1998 at the age of 71; author

"Writing has always helped me through tough times. I began keeping a diary about my experience. It helped to get thoughts – both good and bad – out of my head. Often it let me see that something wasn't as bad as I thought, or it simply organised the thoughts that kept running randomly through my head."
Val Long; diagnosed in 1999 at the age of 47; administrative assistant

"I started writing in my diary for an hour every day. I call it 'My Healing Diary'. I also meditate and take long walks. I have started acupuncture and acupressure treatments to balance my energy and unclog any stagnant areas, and I take Chinese herbs twice daily in the form of tea."
Sandy Rodgers; diagnosed in 1999 at the age of 44; housewife, mother, nurse, Reiki master

"A friend gave me a 'grateful diary' in which to write down my thoughts. I began to write three things I was grateful for each

night. I would drift off to sleep thinking of those things, rather than of the fear that I felt."
Cheryl Cavallo; diagnosed in 1997 at the age of 35; housewife

"I joined a memoir-writing class specifically for breast cancer survivors. That has helped me deal with the emotional impact of having breast cancer."
Judith Ormond; diagnosed in 1996 at the age of 49; symphony musician – piccolo

"I continued to work, and since I am in a helping profession, it was great for me to not have time to dwell on my own problem too much. I did contact a professional colleague and went back into short-term counselling. Of course, I am a three- to five-book-a-week romance reader, which also helped!
Nancie Watson; diagnosed in 1995 at the age of 50; social worker

"I found that a wonderful aid was a pillow speaker, so that I could hear the radio when I woke up startled, remembering that the cancer was real. The small speaker rests on the pillow and distracts you from frightening thoughts. The sound of the radio also helps put you to sleep."
Debbie MacLean; diagnosed in 1991 at the age of 47; volunteer, hospital gift shop and hospice

"My home is my sanctuary. Being able to stay where I choose means I'm in control."
Carrie Drake; diagnosed in 1998 at the age of 42; administrative assistant

"Take care of something. Buy some plants and keep them in good shape. Get a kitten and give it loving attention. The presence of living, growing things at a time of great stress helps decrease the stress and gives you realities outside yourself and your immediate situation. The same thing is true of art. Go to the theatre, a museum, a concert or ballet. Art can take us out of ourselves, lift us beyond our immediate environment, enrich us spiritually and aesthetically. Opening yourself to great beauty is always a life-enhancer. In times of crisis, it's also healing."
Susan Stamberg; diagnosed in 1986 at the age of 48; journalist

"I had two Siamese kittens at the time, and they certainly kept my spirits up. Always an animal lover, I feel that the love of a pet is something everyone should experience."
Barbara C. Sumner; diagnosed in 1982 at the age of 59; housewife

"Before, during and after my mastectomy and reconstruction, I used a series of self-help audiotapes. I think it was due to these tapes that I was able to leave the hospital after a day and a half, rather than the five days predicted. I later used them to relax and programme my body to heal and to handle pain. Turning off the telephone, closing my bedroom door and putting on my earphones was a wonderful escape from the stresses and anxieties of my life. I still use the tapes occasionally now to relax, boost my mood and direct my energies towards healing. Since my diagnosis, I have cured myself of a lifelong eating disorder, quit a job that I hated, fulfilled a lifelong dream by buying a house on the coast and learned an awful lot about love."
Sandra Miller; diagnosed in 1997 at the age of 50; lawyer

"It's important to feel positive and in control during chemo. Have projects to look forward to completing: take computer classes at a local college, do a cross-stitch sampler for a friend's new baby, keep a diary, take watercolour classes. I redecorated my bathroom – I figured I was spending so much time in there, I might as well make it cheerful and fun!"
Sue Braun; diagnosed in 1988 at the age of 41; housewife

"I was diagnosed with cancer in 1978. I had opened a gift and gourmet shop the previous year and was enjoying its success. I am glad I had the shop to keep me busy and my mind from dwelling on the negative."
Adelaide D. Key; diagnosed in 1978 at the age of 42; community volunteer, philanthropist

"After you decide that you're going to live, it's time to make changes for yourself. Do things you want to do and learn how to say 'no' to things you don't. I turned down the chance of being secretary of my local kennel club again. On the other hand, I've become more active in the union at my job. I've also made changes to my lifestyle. For example, I'm now a member of 'our lady of perpetual diets' and I've taken up the treadmill. I really hate this stuff, but I've figured out a way to make it bearable. I'm rewarding myself for weight loss – with jewellery. I have rewards for each weight goal. There's nothing like positive reinforcement to get you to do what's good for you!"

Sharon Irons Strempski; diagnosed in 1997 at the age of 52; nurse

"The best thing I did was decide to take off the rest of the school year and use the time to enjoy my friends and do things I normally didn't have time for. I played with my dog's litter of puppies, met friends for lunch and generally enjoyed my 'holiday'. As I see it, you have two choices: you can put your head under a pillow and go 'Poor me!' or you can get on with your life. I guess you know which I chose."

Lynne Rutenberg; diagnosed in 1980 at the age of 35; retired teacher

Working at It

"At first, I just wanted to stay at home and nurse my wounds, both physical and mental, but I really couldn't. I was running a doctor's office by myself, since my colleague had just moved. My daughter had got engaged a few months before and we were smack in the middle of planning a big wedding. And my husband and I had bought a new house just before my diagnosis, so we had to pack up and move. All great things, but horrible timing! The point of this is that everything worked out fine and the time went by quickly because I was so busy. I was definitely distracted from thinking about cancer!"

Deborah Lambert; diagnosed in 2000 at the age of 47; medical secretary

"My treatment took place in October, November and December – the most stressful time of year. I had to learn to let go of what wasn't important and that included a lot of self-induced stress over the holiday preparations."

Deb Haney; diagnosed in 1996 at the age of 48; administrative assistant, artist

"To keep my spirits up when I wasn't feeling well, I had a quote hanging on my mirror. Muhammad Ali once said, 'I hated every minute of training, but I said to myself, *Suffer now and live the rest of your life as a champion.*' I changed it around to say, 'I hated every

minute of chemo, but I said to myself, *Suffer now and live the rest of your life as a champion.*' "
Asha Mevlana; diagnosed in 1999 at the age of 24; musician

"Before my diagnosis, I had been discouraged by the prospect of turning 50 with my life not going the way I wanted it to. After my surgery, I lay on the couch feeling even worse! I don't know what it was – probably all the phone calls, flowers and cards – but it suddenly hit me. I realised that I could either dwell on this and be miserable or get on with my life. The things I was depressed about were not important. The things I was looking for were right in front of me, and I didn't know it! I had the love of family, friends and colleagues, and most of all my boyfriend Jerry. I am really thankful."
Sharon Daniels; diagnosed in 2000 at the age of 49; hairdresser, wig shop owner

"Because I wanted a full-length bathroom mirror
I had a shower door installed with one
Before I went somewhere, I could check my clothes
See if I looked OK.
Finally, the doctor said I could shower
All of my things gathered, I went in
Started to undress, suddenly, I felt sick
That huge mirror, I was standing in front of it
Without the bandage, I hadn't seen the scar
Didn't want to see it, never wanted to see
That area again. What to do?
A large towel, I hung it over the door,
Covered the mirror. For several months I did that
One day I felt I could look, slowly took the towel down
Crying, I stood there, but realized it didn't look so bad . . .
It has been seven years
I don't think about all these things much any more
Alive, I'm just happy to be
Just to be happy, I'm alive."
Regina Vaughn; diagnosed in 1993 at the age of 45; drapery shop owner

"Hindsight can be harmful. Let go of the 'what ifs', the 'maybes' and the 'should haves'. Practise living life to the full."
Stella Norman; diagnosed in 1999 at the age of 64; addictions counsellor

"My entire being seemed to change overnight. I was no longer the blonde, athletic, zestful, happy-go-lucky girl I'd once been. My past was over, my future looked grim and my present seemed futile. I became so miserable that I was forced to live moment by moment instead of one day at a time. But those moments kept coming, and gradually, like a thousand dazzling lights slow-dancing towards me, I saw that life does go on for cancer patients. This revelation surprised me and filled me with a sense of relief the likes of which I've never felt before. It was as if a great big 'Whew!' blew through me. I began getting up every morning, putting on make-up and getting dressed. One day I accepted an invitation to lunch. Another day I began to take regular walks. Before I knew it, I was back to my old self – except for one major difference. I took nothing for granted – not a star, not a song, not a smile – nothing. Life would never be the same for me. I could grieve or I could celebrate. The choice was mine."
Sallie Burdine; diagnosed in 1998 at the age of 44; author

"I was the only person who could take control of my life. I knew that I was not ready to go anywhere, since I wanted to see my grandchildren grow up. So, after the upset of learning I had cancer, I decided that my humour, my faith and most of all my attitude would help me take control."
Barbara Moro; diagnosed in 1999 at the age of 57; legal secretary

Imagery and Art

"I like visualisation and imagery. It's something that I always put in the category of don't-know-if-it-helps-but-it-can't-hurt! When I was undergoing radiotherapy, I visualised myself sitting under a waterfall in Hawaii and having the water flow over me and wash away all the cancer cells. It was peaceful and calm, and the scenery was beautiful. A couple of times, when the radiotherapist came back into the room and told me I could go, I said I hadn't finished my visualisation, so I couldn't leave just yet!"
Sheilah Musselman; diagnosed in 1997 at the age of 56; nurse

"Years ago, I had heard about the use of visualisation in the treatment of cancer. So I started visualising my healthy 'good' cells travelling through my body wearing 'headlights' like coal miners.

Shining their light beams to identify 'bad' cancer cells, the 'good' cells used picks and shovels to dump the 'bad' cells outside my body. I sent in as many 'good' cells as were needed, until all the 'bad' cancer cells were gone. I still periodically send in those 'good' cells, searching with their 'headlights' to keep my body cancer-free."
Joan Eldredge; diagnosed in 1998 at the age of 65; travel enthusiast, retired psychotherapist

"As an artist I have a vehicle through which I can transform my experiences into healing objects. For instance, when I was in pre-op for surgery, lying there with wires sticking out of my breast to mark the perimeter of my tumour, my surgeon stuck his head in and asked if I was picking up any good radio stations with my antenna. Later I used polymer clay to make a 'boob pin', depicting the breast as an old-fashioned radio, with wire antennas and nipple knobs. I made a smaller 'A cup' size one for the surgeon and a slightly larger 'B cup' size one for myself. For years, I displayed this pin when I did art festivals as a reminder to women to have regular mammograms and to the men in their lives to see that they did."
Jeanne Sturdevant; diagnosed in 1990 at the age of 45; artist

"I was first diagnosed in 1978, a divorced single mother of 38. For the better part of 22 years, I have lived with breast cancer, and life is joyful, precious and peaceful. Because I am a collagist, I favour the 'collage approach' to coping. A collage is an art form in which diverse elements are arranged to form a new image. Collage is also an empowering metaphor for designing life. Each of us is the powerful creator of the work of art in progress – the masterpiece known as our life. The elements in my own personal collage include twice-daily meditation, regular yoga practice, a vegetarian diet, therapeutic massages, sessions with a hands-on energy healer, time spent in the country, reading, reading, reading, writing and making collages. I coach people in using the latter – a simple tool for releasing stress and upsets, discovering one's true Self and learning the pleasure of creative expression. My home is a sanctuary filled with delights for all my senses. I cultivate quiet, calm, contemplation, close friendships and love. I consciously practise a 'gratitude attitude' daily, count my many blessings and make certain that each day is as delicious as I can make it."
Susan Zimmerman; diagnosed in 1978 at the age of 38; collagist

"The Worry Box"

"I found that the most constructive thing I did was to say, 'I have cancer.' Like many people, I didn't want to say the word. It was like swearing in front of a priest! I also had to tell my family that it was okay to say 'cancer'. It is important to be able to say it freely. It is also important to let people know that you are not giving up on life. I was not going to let cancer get me down. I refused to worry about it. I knew that worrying wouldn't help and that positive thinking was important. Attitude has a lot to do with your recuperation."
Barbara Moro; diagnosed in 1999 at the age of 57; legal secretary

"I think one of the very best things I did was to talk about what I was going through. I told everyone I could. Saying the words 'I've been diagnosed with breast cancer' helped me accept my situation. I didn't want people to feel weird talking to me after they found out from others. Telling them myself meant they were able to see that I was okay. I think that my honesty and openness gave me strength and had a big impact on my friends and family. I tried to keep the tone light, positive and upbeat when I talked to people, and this made them want to stay connected to me. I needed this connection, and I needed it on a daily basis. I needed to hear myself sounding okay."
Julie Crandall; diagnosed in 1998 at the age of 31; housewife and mother

"Talk, talk, talk. The more you talk about your problems, the more people around you will understand what you're going through. They are going through this with you, too."
Tammi Keller; diagnosed in 2000 at the age of 30; mother

"One of the things that helped me get through this was talking to friends and family about my feelings and concerns. One friend advised me to take charge of my illness, not to leave it up to other people. I truly believe this is one reason why I have been cancer-free for 13 years."
Polly Briggs; diagnosed in 1987 at the age of 41; secretary

"When I felt depressed, I went for counselling. It was the best thing I could have done. I learned to love myself – a very important part of the healing process."
E. Mary Lou Clauss; diagnosed in 1991 at the age of 55; retired nurse

"See a counsellor. I did, and it helped relieve my anxiety and my feeling of hopelessness. It was a very positive experience."
Rhonda Sorrell; diagnosed in 1998 at the age of 43; special needs teacher

"Plan a trip now for a post-treatment celebration. It will give you something to look forward to."
Alexandra Koffman; diagnosed in 1997 at the age of 40; nurse

"The best advice I got was from a good friend who said, 'Pamper yourself! If it feels good, do it!' That sometimes meant a good cry and a long nap."
Sharon Carr; diagnosed in 1997 at the age of 42; hospice grief counsellor

"Allow yourself life's little indulgences. It feels good. Indulge in a good cry when you need it."
Susan Rothstein; diagnosed in 1997 at the age of 49; travel agent

"The Worry Box. In the winter of 1992, when I was 42, I was diagnosed with breast cancer. I was immediately focused. I knew what I had to do, and I did it. I researched my disease, and my family and I made decisions. After the mastectomy, though, I began to worry. I worried about our decisions and the impact of all that had happened on my family. I worried about the future. I worried about a recurrence. I worried about my daughter. I worried about *everything*. A counsellor suggested a strategy that helped me more than anything. I found a box and glued colourful scraps of wrapping paper on the top. Inside it, each morning, I tucked handwritten notes about my worries and fears. Then I closed the lid and went on with the rest of the day, whether it was walking in the woods, listening to music, grocery shopping, paying bills or cuddling up with my daughter to read a book. The Worry Box also provided me with a concrete way of saying 'Enough! I want to live my life and make the most of each and every day!' I have the box to this day."
Nancy Burgess; diagnosed in 1992 at the age of 42; teacher, mother, wife

"Do things for other people. There are always people who are worse off than you are. It takes your mind off your own troubles."
Betty Pollom; daughter of Frances Davis

7 · Family

Our Inheritance

amily members come with the territory. We don't ask to have them. We're born, and they're there. In the old days, we lived on the same street, if not in the same house with them, even into adulthood – and in some instances that hasn't changed. More often, though, they now live on the other side of town, even at the other end of the country. They may not be involved in our lives on a daily basis, until something like breast cancer hits. Then they gather round in person, on the phone or over the Web.

How many times have we said – or overheard others say – what a shame that it takes a crisis to bring families together? So why does that happen? Is it because of a shared past, shared memories? Is it because of a shared gene pool, which means other family members immediately have an investment in the disease? Is it because, deep down, when we move past extreme expectations and consequent disappointments, sibling rivalry and petty grievances, we feel a primal link?

A family is a support group. It isn't necessarily the kind of support group that gives you answers, but rather the kind that is there to help. But here we go again with those extreme expectations. We assume that our family will know just what we need. Unfortunately, that isn't always true. This may be our relatives' first experience with breast cancer, and watching us go through it may be harder than if they were going through it themselves. We need to tell them what we need, but that is sometimes easier said than done.

"There are times when I feel that no one wants to talk to me about my cancer," writes Glenda Chance, a wife and mother who was diagnosed in 2000 at the age of 38. "How do I get my loved ones to understand that even though it is a painful subject, it is a subject that I need to talk about? I am not looking for them to give me the right answers or even say all the right things. They just need to know that just because my body has healed after the operation, my mind and heart have not. But . . . it's me. I'm at fault, too. I've created a silence and used it to push them away. It's up to me to involve them in my life and tell them how I feel. They, too, are survivors in this, and they need to know from us what they can do to make our lives easier."

Yes, they need to know what they can do, but they also need to know that we want their help. Carol Englund, who was diagnosed in 1994 at the age of 58, writes, "I truly believe that without my family, I would not have come as easily to the place where I am now. As important as it is for us to be able to accept the help of others, it is also important for them to know that they *can* help."

This chapter is a step in that direction. It's a small step, a tentative one, given that one woman's family situation may be very different from another's. But it's a starting point. Just as our families have a disproportionate power to disappoint, so they can also boost us in wondrous ways.

And the boosting can go on for years. As survivor Debbie MacLean wrote, "Where did I hear about *UPLIFT*? My son Douglas sent me a card on the tenth anniversary of my being diagnosed!"

When I First Learned . . .

"The most difficult person to tell about my diagnosis was my mother. She lives a long way away. We only see each other once or twice a year. Fortunately, she had planned to come for a visit soon after I was diagnosed, so I was able to tell her in person and she could see that I was doing all right. She did not come for the surgery, which was my family's choice. The day of my operation, my sister-in-law's mother turned up unannounced at Mother's with a huge picnic lunch (in January!), and she spent the day with my

mother until my husband called to say everything had gone smoothly. I always felt that was one of the most generous gifts anyone could have given my mother that day. Isabelle knew my mother would be worried, and she did her best to provide her with some company and cheer her up."
Wanda Null; diagnosed in 1986 at the age of 41; librarian

"It was hardest to tell my mum. She has gone through some great sadness in her life, and she has always been a pillar of strength. I needed her in my corner for that very reason. The news spread through my family quickly, and I went on to tell my children's teachers and my friends and colleagues. Telling all these people helped me to be in charge."
Cindy Fiedler; diagnosed in 1998 at the age of 40; nurse, mother

"Telling my mum, who lived 800 miles away, was tough. My dad died 18 years ago from brain cancer and now I had to tell her I had cancer. That was a very hard phone call, but she was there for me and came to be by my side."
Kathy Rabassa; diagnosed in 1999 at the age of 34; administrative assistant

"When I first found out I had breast cancer, my in-laws were living a long way away. My mother-in-law was so supportive. She told me that if I needed to talk, just to call her. She might not understand a word I was saying, but she was there to listen. My brother-in-law called me after each treatment just to ask 'how you all are'. That meant so much to me. As a special thank you, I baked him a raspberry pie (his favourite)."
Nancy Ellis; diagnosed in 2000 at the age of 53; quality control technician

"I feared most telling my parents that their oldest daughter had cancer. We don't live in the same area and I couldn't break the news on the phone, so I wrote them a letter. I made it clear that what I needed most was their love, support and optimism. They called within a day of receiving my letter and were very positive."
Carrie Drake; diagnosed in 1998 at the age of 42; administrative assistant

"I most feared telling my parents, so I told them last. I went to their home early in the morning, sat at the kitchen table with them and

spoke in reference to my father's mother. 'You know how Nana had varicose veins, and I have them, too. And you know how Nana had bunions, and I have them, too. I seem to have her breast cancer as well.' As always, my father took control. He wanted to make arrangements for the two of us to fly thousands of miles to take advantage of the latest treatments. I declined. I hate flying."
Deborah J. P. Schur; diagnosed in 1994 at the age of 43; sales rep

"My daughter and I did not get along well before this, but when I had cancer, she changed dramatically. She said, 'I will be here to take care of you,' and she was."
Barbara Moro; diagnosed in 1999 at the age of 57; legal secretary

"When I first learned I had breast cancer, I only told two people: my husband and my best friend. My three sons were away at college and in the midst of final exams. I didn't want to give them any news that would distract them from their studies. Then, on the last day of radiotherapy, they and their girlfriends sent me a large bouquet of flowers. The poor delivery man had to wait until I stopped crying before he could leave."
Fran Hegarty; diagnosed in 2000 at the age of 47; librarian

"The best thing I did after learning of my diagnosis was to keep the news between my husband and myself. We did the Christmas holidays as planned, so that they could be enjoyed before the family knew of my upcoming surgery."
Irene Louise; diagnosed in 1995 at the age of 41; retired executive secretary

"A cancer diagnosis can bring out of people an openness and honesty that is so genuine. One of the most touching moments I experienced after I was diagnosed was when my brother called me to talk. He said that he had been thinking about me and crying, which in itself was a shock, because I hadn't seen him cry since we were kids. We were talking about the cancer, and he said, 'I love you, Jules . . .' Although we have always been very close, we had never said 'I love you' to each other before. It was a very special moment. I still get a little choked up when I think about it. When there is a cancer diagnosis, there is an urgency to express our feelings, and that is how it should be. It is important to help everyone realise how

special they are. When someone is facing a serious illness, there is no greater gift than those simple words, 'I love you, Jules . . .' "
Julie Crandall; diagnosed in 1998 at the age of 31; housewife and mother

Telling the Kids

"When I was diagnosed with breast cancer, the hardest thing for me was to tell my son, who was ten at the time. In the three preceding years, we had lost several family members to cancer. He didn't know anyone who had survived, or so he thought. I pointed out to him that his grandmother and an aunt had breast cancer many years ago, and here they are today."
Tammy Delin; diagnosed in 1997 at the age of 33; teacher's assistant

"My family had bad feelings about radiotherapy because of my father's illness. There was tension and fear. So I insisted that my children, their spouses and my two grandchildren come with me to radiotherapy to see what it was about. As they did I could feel the tension leave their bodies. What the mind imagines is far worse than reality. My eight-year-old granddaughter said, 'Grandma, what's the big deal? We see you lying that way on your bed!' My daughter Karen, who was 34 when I went through my treatment, says that the more open I was with my feelings, the better it was for her. She lives near me and appreciated going to see where the radiotherapy took place. That way she could picture it and it wasn't the gloomy thing she had imagined."
Anne Jacobs; diagnosed in 1999 at the age of 62; managing partner, estate agency

"I was concerned about my grandson seeing me without any hair. He was just turning two and had always held on to the side of my hair to fall asleep. One afternoon, it was so hot that I took my wig off and laid it on the back of the couch. He came in, sat beside me, and pointed to the wig. 'Is that your hair?' he asked. I told him that it was, and he told me to put it back on and laughed. After that I knew I didn't have to wear that wig all day long."
Carol Keen; diagnosed in 1999 at the age of 48; office clerk

"My daughter was 15, frightened and depressed. She had a wonderful history teacher who took her aside and disclosed that she

was a survivor and shared her and her family's experiences. It
made all the difference."
Barbara Jentis; diagnosed in 1983 at the age of 41; lawyer

"Allow your children to help you. My 16-year-old daughter blos-
somed right in front of my eyes. She thrived on helping me with
the housework and the cooking, along with her younger sister,
with whom she became very close. She grew tremendously in self-
confidence and self-esteem."
Cornelia Doherty; diagnosed in 1985 at the age of 45; mother, widow,
speaker

"My children were eight and 14 at the time, and the younger one
handled it much better than the older one. My older daughter was
concerned that we had not told her all the details. So we invited
her to accompany us to the hospital when we went for a second
opinion. The day of my operation she missed school and kept her
father company at the hospital."
Wanda Null; diagnosed in 1986 at the age of 41; librarian

"The most humbling experience I had with breast cancer was having my son, a nurse, take care of my incision and drainage tubes
after my operation."
Rosamary Amiet; diagnosed in 2000 at the age of 48; programme
manager

"My husband and son were very, very good to me. My son used to
joke around and keep me laughing, even though he was scared
himself. One day, when he wanted me to go somewhere with him,
he said, 'Put your wig on, sister, and let's go!' He told me that I
didn't need to go to a support group, that I had a support group at
home, and he was right. My son is 20."
Paula Porter; diagnosed in 2000 at the age of 47; telephone operator

"When I had to spend several weeks in hospital, away from my children, a friend gave me a wonderful suggestion. I brought loads of
small 'prizes' – stickers, key rings, rubbers, pencils and so on. I
wrote short notes and enclosed a prize with each note. I prepared
lots of these pre-packaged prizes and took them along with me
to the hospital. Every day, when my husband visited, I sent an

envelope home with him for each child. It made me feel connected to each child every day, even when I felt too weak to talk on the phone. I think my children were almost disappointed when I came home!"

Vivian; diagnosed in 1998 at the age of 36; professor

"My son, who was 14 when I was diagnosed, remembers feeling disbelief. He says that what gave him the most comfort was my keeping him informed of the status of my health and treatments. My 12-year-old son understood my need to rest on the day of a treatment and kept his friends quiet while they played in the house. The day the dressing came off my incision, he ran into the house and asked to see it. I held up my shirt. He took a long hard look, and went back outdoors to play, seemingly content that everything looked fine. My daughter, who was not quite nine when I was diagnosed, went to school the next day and quite matter-of-factly told her art teacher that I had breast cancer. I think the teacher was floored!"

Deborah J. P. Schur; diagnosed in 1994 at the age of 43; sales rep

"My diagnosis of breast cancer was the most shocking experience of my life. My husband's mum had died of breast cancer when he was 30, and it brought up many emotions for both of us. But he said to me, 'It looks as if we have a battle to fight, and we are going to win.' He was my 'knight in shining armour' – there for me, supporting me, taking care of me and the kids every step of the way. We have three children. Our girl was 14, and our boys were eight and two and a half. We told them the truth from the beginning and answered all of their questions honestly. I made sure that our daughter knew that she wasn't expected to take on my household responsibilities. We had friends help me, so that she didn't have any additional burdens in her already busy life. She also made a positive affirmation about her breasts growing, so that her fear wouldn't affect it. As for me, I got a nutritionist and cleaned up my already fairly healthy, predominantly organic food diet as much as I could. I went on a cleansing diet first, which helped a lot before my surgery and chemo."

Sandy Rodgers; diagnosed in 1999 at the age of 44; housewife, mother nurse, Reiki master

With Me Every Step of the Way

"My son and his wife made arrangements to have my house cleaned during my recovery from surgery. It wasn't that the cleaning itself was so important to me, but that they had thought to do this for me."
Susan Smith; diagnosed in 2000 at the age of 53; medical library technician

"My mother, grandmother, Aunt Dee and Aunt Judy (my godmother, who travelled hundreds of miles to be here) cleaned my house from top to bottom and then polished all of the leaves on my house plants with mayonnaise!!"
Beth Compton; diagnosed in 1995 at the age of 27; civil engineer

"My grandmother sent me a cheque with instructions that I was to have fresh flowers in the house at all times. I love flowers, but usually splurge on them only for special occasions, so having them around for months on end felt like a special treat. It was a soul-nourishing gift, especially since I was diagnosed in the middle of a long bleak winter."
Dorian Solot; diagnosed in 2000 at the age of 26

"My family helped me considerably, financially as well as physically. They even bought me a new sofa and chair so that I could be comfortable on those days when I didn't feel well. My mum and two sisters travelled over several times to spend time with me. It was wonderful having them there as a support system and also, during my surgery, knowing that they were at my home taking care of everything and my two cats. It was one less thing to think about."
Gwen Loverink; diagnosed in 1994 at the age of 34; police dispatcher

"The most special thing that was done for me was that my older brother wrote me a cheque for the amount of money I had made before my diagnosis for the entire year. He didn't want me to think about losing money from not working. All he wanted me to do was to concentrate on getting better!"
Cathy Hanlon; diagnosed in 2000 at the age of 42; school researcher

"The most practical things my family did to help? Several family

members sent money. Others had a stackable washer/dryer installed for me."
Carrie Drake; diagnosed in 1998 at the age of 42; administrative assistant

"One of my daughters made a countdown calendar for me, starting with six and going down to zero. I tacked it to my bathroom door and after each chemo treatment I tore off a page. What a sense of triumph it was to tear off those pages one at a time before finally reaching the last one."
Faye Hardiman; diagnosed in 1998 at the age of 50; wife, mother, teacher

"Friends or family members can help by taping videos of great upbeat romantic comedies – e.g., *Sleepless in Seattle, When Harry Met Sally* – for you to watch while recovering from treatment. They can also prepare meals and freeze them for future consumption. Receiving phone calls from friends and family is the best medicine."
Ellen Beth Simon; diagnosed in 1998 at the age of 41; lawyer

"The most practical thing done for me by a family member was when my mother-in-law did my laundry."
Frances Gallello; diagnosed in 2000 at the age of 51; mental health assistant

"My son Michael brought me a Cabbage Patch doll. The doll went with me to all my doctor's appointments. My surgeon's comment when he saw the doll was, 'You pull out all the stops, don't you!' "
Jeryl Abelmann; diagnosed in 1986 at the age of 46; primary school teacher

"My one niece, Suzanne, knew the right questions to ask the surgeon. Questions, questions, questions. Do not be afraid to ask!"
Barbara Moro; diagnosed in 1999 at the age of 57; legal secretary

"My sister Vel, who lives a long way away, was phoning all the time and sending cards daily, plus surprise packages. She made every effort to let me know that she was there for me. She's a true blessing in my life."
Sherry Ann Wells; diagnosed in 1997 at the age of 45; housewife

"I felt empowered by the goodness of people. My sister travelled for 16 hours by train to see me. She did not come alone but brought her infant son, and she did it numerous times. She cleaned my house, did my laundry and talked to me for hours about the things only sisters can talk about. She gave me hope. My mother insisted on driving me to every session of chemotherapy and radiotherapy. Not that I wasn't perfectly capable of doing it myself, but she indicated that this was not optional. My Aunt Chris provided me with an endless supply of homemade chicken soup. This helped me do battle with the nausea that I felt during chemotherapy. Friends and family members called and sent flowers, sweets and even money."
Cindy Fiedler; diagnosed in 1998 at the age of 40; nurse, mother

"Above all else, I was fortunate to have my husband sitting next to me for 11 months during my treatments."
Susan Schultz; diagnosed in 1990 at the age of 41; special needs teacher's assistant

"When my husband and I bought a new house in the middle of my chemotherapy treatments, my cousin and brother-in-law packed us up and moved us, and my sister unpacked and organised my kitchen and bedroom when I couldn't get off the sofa."
Linda Perkins; diagnosed in 1999 at the age of 35; project manager

"During my stem cell treatment, I was not allowed to see my children for two weeks and I found that devastating. However, my husband formed his game plan for the toughest game of our lives. He stayed in the hospital isolation room with me for the entire two-week period, except for when he attended my daughter's university basketball game and the pageant in which she was a contestant."
Fran DiBiase; diagnosed in 1994 at the age of 40; part-time teacher, part-time property management executive

"I knew I would be recovering from my surgery for four to six weeks. My husband, who is the absolute greatest, cannot cook. He only defrosts. So I spent a couple of days before surgery cooking our favourite meals and putting them in single-serving cartons and freezing them. The cooking was therapeutic for me, and we ate well for quite a while!"
Jennifer Wersal; diagnosed in 2000 at the age of 30; marketing executive

"My family has been there for me every step of the way, making sure that the everyday chores are taken care of, that I am properly nourished, and just being very supportive in everything they do and say. Since my diagnosis, my youngest daughter has even undertaken to do breast cancer research at her school!"
Carol Downer; diagnosed in 1997 at the age of 48; legal secretary

When My Mum Was Diagnosed . . .

"Having my mum diagnosed with breast cancer was a life-defining event for me. I was 29 at the time and filled with my life's happenings, and I had taken her presence for granted. I attended every doctor's appointment with her, and when she had a mastectomy, I was blessed to be able to give back a small fraction of the care and love that she had given me for so many years. We were together on the day she received the news that her cancer had not spread. Before she was diagnosed, we had started planning a cruise to the Bahamas with friends. That cruise became her celebration of life – even though she worried that she would lose her prosthesis in the ocean. I don't think that I have ever told her, but her strength and positive attitude through it all blew me away."
Jennifer Schuster; daughter of a survivor

"Breast cancer can devastate a person's health, yet all the while encourage the soul to bloom. When my family was told of my mother's diagnosis, our hearts seemed to stop. I cried more tears then than I had in my lifetime. Yet, my mother's touch was peaceful and accepting. Over the past nine months, she has experienced pain, but she remains strong. She is determined to conquer this cancer – not with shouts of anger, but by providing unconditional love to hurting friends and family and gentle words of hope to those who support her. In my mind, she has already won."
Heather Marie Zielke; daughter of a survivor

"I remember getting a call from my mum, and her giving me the bad news that she had just been diagnosed with breast cancer. She was so upbeat that I remember thinking she must be in shock. As the months passed and she went through chemo treatments, she paid close attention to her diet and exercised on a regular basis. She still seemed too happy to me. I kept wondering how I'd feel if

I were in her shoes, and the only word that came to mind was 'devastated'. Yet, there Mum was, laughing and checking up to see how
everyone else was doing. Never once did I see her cry. Well, she
won! She has now been cancer-free for a while. To this day, she has
neither cried nor shown self-pity. The main thing this has shown
me is that my mother has an inner strength the likes of which I
never knew existed. That strength, along with faith and the grace
of God, can lead us through anything in life."
Bec Wiget; daughter of a survivor

"In the busy times we live in, we don't always have the ability to see
our family members every day. My mother's chemotherapy treatment required injections for ten consecutive days after each treatment. For those ten days, over a period of months, I would inject
my mum, sit at the kitchen table and chat with my mum and grandmother. The positive side was a retreat back to times when families
visited each other every day!"
Regina R. Young; daughter of Claire E. Reber

"On a visit to my mum when she was having chemo, I did her nails.
She enjoyed that so much. My massaging her hands and filing and
polishing her nails was very relaxing to her. I think it's important
for women going through this to be good to themselves – whether
it's having their nails done or their hair washed, or doing something else that is relaxing and fun."
Laura Thomas; daughter of Roberta Price Wilcox

"My sister Cathleen is my best friend. We are 14 months apart in
age and have always been close. She was diagnosed, against all sta-
tistics, before she was 30. To say that we were shocked is an under-
statement. I am doing as much as I can to support her and offer an
ear or a shoulder whenever she needs it. And her two littlest
angels, my sons Seth and Benjamin, are two of her strongest life-
lines."
Angela Thompson; sister of Cathleen D'Antonio

"How do you comfort someone you love who has been told she has
breast cancer? What words can ease the fear? How can you help
her sleep at night? Reading! Books have a way of taking you into
another world, time and place. I gave Nan one of my favourite

books and told her that even if she just read a few pages at night, it would help her. Today, my sister reads about eight books a month. She also belongs to a book group. She says that I've given her the gift of reading, and what a pot of gold that is!"
Maybelle Timm Eley; sister of Nan Comstock

"Humour and a strong faith in God were two of the most important tools that helped our family make it through a terrifying time. My mother-in-law is a breast cancer survivor today, and we are so very grateful. We constantly teased her about her bald head and even about her lopsided chest. I know that might seem distasteful to some, but we chose to smile rather than walk about looking stricken. The loss of her breast was traumatic, but it was such a small part of a wonderful woman who is so much more than any breast can be!"
Judi Scally; daughter-in-law of Marian Scally

"I was totally untouched by breast cancer until my favourite aunt developed it two years ago, shortly before my son's wedding. She wanted to make sure that she had the necessary surgery in time to enjoy the wedding, so that her absence didn't put a damper on the festivities. Because of a bad cold and several other mishaps, the date of her surgery kept being delayed. She finally had the operation just two weeks before the wedding, but still she was determined to be with us. Though she'd had the option of staying in private homes, she insisted on staying at the hotel so that everyone got to see her at the big party my husband and I held there the night before the wedding. She wanted to make sure that she would see everyone then and answer all their questions, so the focus the next night would be on the bride and groom alone. Well, on the night of the wedding, everybody was in a party mood, and there was my Aunt Jean, up on the dance floor celebrating with everyone else! I know she was in pain, but she let nothing stop her or *any* of us from enjoying a very special event!"
Marilyn Eichner; niece of Jean Firkser

Among My Cancer Blessings . . .

"Among my cancer blessings were spending a great deal of cherished time with my husband as he took time off from work, finding

out that I look pretty good with very short hair and realising the amazing trust my two teenagers had in me when I said, 'The doctors are going to take care of me. I'm going to be okay.' "
Diane Bongiorno; diagnosed in 1998 at the age of 43; instructional aide

"My kids were great; they did a million things to bolster my spirits, as did my husband. My daughter did a breast cancer walk in my honour. The sight of her crossing the finish line will always be a cherished moment."
Suzanne Pollock; diagnosed in 1995 at the age of 50; stationer

"Support and love and laughter from the Ablemenn in my life brought me the strength I needed to get through this time of my life."
Jeryl Abelmann; diagnosed in 1986 at the age of 46; primary school teacher

"Friends and family need to keep panic in check. When my close cousin in Israel e-mailed me her hysteria, I told her that I couldn't correspond that way. And it stopped."
Anne Jacobs; diagnosed in 1999 at the age of 62; managing partner, estate agency

"I became twins with my bald dad. We had numerous photos taken like that."
Asha Mevlana; diagnosed in 1999 at the age of 24; musician

"During chemotherapy treatments, some weekends I felt much better than others. My husband and I always made simple plans for those weekends, apple picking or taking a walk on the beach. On my bad weekends, our family took comfort from just talking and being together. A family celebration fell during one of my more difficult chemotherapy treatments. As a family, we decided to move it to a different date. It gave us something to plan for and look forward to."
Helaine Hemingway; diagnosed in 1988 at the age of 41; teacher

"I have just celebrated my two-year survivor anniversary. I was diagnosed when my daughter was four months old and had had bilateral mastectomies by the time she turned five months old. It

was an eye-opening experience for my husband and me, particularly since we had been married only a year and a half when this occurred. We are expecting our second child this summer, and truly feel that our children are miracles. Our first child was a miracle because if I hadn't had her I would have never found the cancer as quickly as I did. Our second is a miracle because we have overcome so much. We didn't know if I would be able to have any more children because I'd had cancer, but when I had my yearly visit with my oncologist, she gave me a clean bill of health."
Tresa Johnson; diagnosed in 1999 at the age of 23; PA

"We booked a holiday. Then I was diagnosed with breast cancer. I kept telling Jerry I couldn't go because of how I would feel after treatments, but he wouldn't hear of our not going. He said he would carry me if he had to, so I could see my son, who had recently moved to the area. Well, we had a great time! A whole crowd of us went – family and friends, even my ex – and there was a big surprise: my daughter and her boyfriend got married there. I wish her health and happiness!"
Sharon Daniels; diagnosed in 2000 at the age of 49; hairdresser, wig shop owner

"My birthday was eight weeks after my diagnosis and my family wanted to take me out to dinner. This was my first real night out since D-day (diagnosis day), and I remember feeling reasonably good and a bit excited about dressing up and going out. I'll never forget going to my bedroom with hopes of finding something pretty to wear. Instead I came out in tears. Nothing in my new beautiful scarf collection matched any of my old not-so-beautiful clothes. All of my scarves were printed and therefore clashed with the majority of my clothes, which were also printed. I needed a new wardrobe. My husband was taken aback when I announced this to him – bald, crying on my birthday, and in front of my parents. But he said, 'Of course, sweetheart, anything you need.' After that, getting dressed became a breeze. Almost as easy as . . . the drop of a hat (had to say it)!"
Sallie Burdine; diagnosed in 1998 at the age of 44; author

"After countless compositions in my head, when I finally sat down to write something that I thought would be profound, I discovered that everything I thought I had to say was totally bland. How could I be an inspiration to anyone? Then I remembered that despite the fact that I was not near family members during my surgery and subsequent treatment and recovery period, I was constantly in touch with them through the magic of e-mail. This is such a wonderful way to keep in touch with the outside world. I received and sent letters on a daily basis, documented my true feelings to family members who I knew would care, wrote short stories and poems for personal satisfaction, and found joy in the many inspirational poems and essays that family members forwarded to me."

Florence Wade; diagnosed in 1999 at the age of 63; retired school teacher, retired property manager

"I was 26, and I had breast cancer. I didn't know how, but I knew why. I got breast cancer because God wanted me to be able to share my experience with other women. Up to this point I still wasn't sure what I wanted to do with my life. My kids were at school, so I had time to do anything I wanted, but I had no idea what that was. The first thing on my agenda was to kick this cancer into touch. Luckily, I had nothing but the best medical care. I went through eight sessions of chemo in six months. I lost my hair, lost weight and gained a whole new respect for myself. I couldn't get over how strong and how happy I was. I grew to love my husband and children more and more every day. I had thought I loved them all that I could. How wrong I was. If you've never stared death in the face and won, then you haven't lived. Every day when I wake up and see my kids' smiling faces and hear those precious words, 'I love you, Mummy,' I get goosepimples. I fell in love with my husband all over again. There I was, thinking I looked like something that the cat had dragged in, and he would tell me how beautiful I was and how much he thanked God that I came into his life."

Kimberlee Richardson; diagnosed in 2000 at the age of 26; mother, air force wife, student

8 • Friends

We Pick 'Em

Not all of us have family. Breast cancer hits women who are single and divorced, who have no siblings and whose parents are no longer alive, who live too far away for their family to help with the mechanics of juggling cancer and life, or who simply . . . don't get on with their family. For these women, friends are their family.

I am fortunate enough to have family *and* friends. No, my problem wasn't having people who would have helped if I'd asked. My problem was asking. Survivors warn against this. They point out, time and again, that people really do want to help and that their help makes all the difference. Another of my problems, of course, was that many friends didn't know I had breast cancer. If they didn't know, how could they cook for me? Or send cards? Or ring up just to let me have a moan?

Lest you start feeling sorry for me, let me say that I wasn't suffering. In addition to my family and those few close friends in the know, I had the characters I was writing about at the time. They were wonderfully solicitous, waiting patiently while I took time off for a treatment, a lunch date, a manicure or a nap. They took me outside myself and my own problems, helped me put things in perspective – because *they* were dealing with Alzheimer's disease. By comparison, I had it easy.

But this chapter isn't about imaginary friends; it's about real ones. If I were to single out the nicest thing that a friend did for me during this period, it would have to be the generosity of Jane.

Months before my mastectomy, I had agreed to speak at a national conference in a city I'd never visited before. Then breast cancer came along, and I had my mastectomy a mere six weeks before the conference. I was fine. I could go. My luggage was the problem. It was heavy.

I was into the saline expansion phase of my reconstruction, and my chest and upper arms were weak. So I brought Jane with me as my own personal porter, and we had a ball. We saw the sights, explored the city, toasted each other at every possible meal. As far as anyone else knew, she had come along just to keep me company – a reasonable excuse, given how lonely business travel is. Bless him, my husband came through even then. When we checked into our hotel, there were roses and chocolate-dipped strawberries waiting for us! Steve knew that I'd been apprehensive about the mechanics of the trip and, unable to get away himself, was as grateful to Jane as I was.

This chapter has two purposes. First, I want women who are newly diagnosed to take a deep breath and realise that they aren't alone, that friends do come through. Second, I want *friends* to be able to glance through these pages, gain a better understanding of survivors' needs and therefore have more of an idea how they can help.

Sometimes that simply means being there and not doing a thing, which brings me to a quick word about the term "friends". I take it in its broadest sense. Hence I give you Bear.

"To help me pass the time," wrote Barbara Moro, a legal secretary, "I went to work, slept when I was really tired and spent time with my best friend, my dog Bear. I know it sounds strange, but he was very soothing to me when I was feeling rough. He was most attentive to me during this time."

I find that humbling. As arrogant as we humans are – as certain that we are a higher species – our pets do sense what we need. In bad times, without a word of instruction from us, they come through. If they were able to speak or to write, I would have solicited their help with this chapter. Instead, I rely on the following very human words.

Breaking the Ice

"As soon as I found out I had breast cancer, I called everyone I

knew so that they would hear it from me directly and not feel weird talking about it with me. I also created a website to document my experiences, so that people who weren't comfortable talking to me about it could learn what I was going through on their own terms. I had so many people calling on the phone that I couldn't keep up with it all. So I changed my answering machine to say: 'If you want to know what's happened to Asha, press 1. If you want to know her treatment plan, press 2. If you want to know how she's doing, press 3.' "
Asha Mevlana; diagnosed in 1999 at the age of 24; musician

"I told everyone that I had breast cancer. I didn't want people talking behind my back. Some people didn't know what to say to me, but I hadn't changed. I was the same person I'd always been."
Judy Peterson; diagnosed in 2000 at the age of 58; nurse

"Actually, I think going out in public helps to break the ice for others. I learned from my experience that others were more frightened than I was about encountering me back in the 'real' world. But once the initial hello and/or hug and/or acknowledgement was over with, so was the awkwardness."
Sallie Burdine; diagnosed in 1998 at the age of 44; author

"During recovery, people were hesitant towards me, not knowing how to react. I quickly realised that they were taking their cue from me. They calmed down when they saw that my reaction was positive."
Carol Pasternak; diagnosed in 1986 at the age of 47; artist

"People often just don't know what to say to you. They try to put emotions into words, and that can't always be done. I always appreciated a simple 'Good luck, we're thinking of you.' "
Kim Vermeire; diagnosed in 1992 at the age of 18; computer consultant

"It is important to understand that some people are *afraid* to speak to you about breast cancer."
Eleanor Anbinder; diagnosed in 1991 at the age of 50; sales manager

"Let people hug you. It warms your sad heart!"
Sarah Stuart; diagnosed in 1999 at the age of 52; banking personnel assistant

"I had always been a very private person who dealt with my own problems and didn't burden others. I opened up to people and discovered how caring they can be when you give them the chance. I am much more open now about things."
Sue Watson; diagnosed in 1996 at the age of 53; teacher

"People were trying to protect me and second-guess me. I think they were more frightened than I was. Of course, I was doing too much and was tired, so I was possibly sending the wrong message."
Sandy Williams; diagnosed in 1999 at the age of 51; children's public librarian

"The best thing I did for myself was to go shopping with a friend. She insisted I buy myself something pretty and comfortable for hospital. We spent all day at the shopping centre. She was wonderfully patient with me."
Fran Hegarty; diagnosed in 2000 at the age of 47; librarian

"What most raised my spirits when my hair started falling out were the friends – both male and female – who often told me I was beautiful."
Carrie Drake; diagnosed in 1998 at the age of 42; administrative assistant

"I cried a lot. I appreciated the people who just listened to me cry."
Suzanne Pollock; diagnosed in 1995 at the age of 50; stationer

"My husband had a business dinner, so I went out with a friend. We talked about her marriage. It was therapy to listen to someone else's challenges in life."
Sandy Williams; diagnosed in 1999 at the age of 51; children's public librarian

"My advice to friends? Listen, listen, listen. Sometimes we need to talk. But talk about your own life, too. We need to be as involved as we ever were with the rest of our lives."
Anne Jacobs; diagnosed in 1999 at the age of 62; managing partner, estate agency

"The most helpful thing others did for me after my diagnosis was to hug me. No words would comfort me, but arms enfolding me

were comforting. In turn, I learned to give hugs to friends and strangers. It's the best!"
Deborah J. P. Schur; diagnosed in 1994 at the age of 43; sales rep

"What I remember most about the first week of diagnosis was the outpouring of support from family and friends. I could have opened up a card shop, a florist's and a restaurant with all the cards, flowers and food that was sent. One of the most touching things that week was returning home from several hours of medical tests to find that my next-door neighbours had cut our grass!"
Beth Compton; diagnosed in 1995 at the age of 27; civil engineer

"Just one day after my operation, I was discharged from hospital. The dark dismal morning mirrored my spirits. I brought my hand up to the bandages that covered my chest and a nurse instructed me on the care of my alien breast. My husband arrived to take me home and we drove in silence. The rain became a steady drizzle as grief tightened its grip. When we pulled into our drive, though, a splash of colour exploded before my eyes. Two newly planted borders framed the path to my house. Pansies, salvia, petunias and impatiens created a kaleidoscope of colour. 'Who?' I asked my husband, but I already knew. 'Eileen, Kate and Cathy,' he said, adding with a smile, 'and in the pouring rain, too.' The next morning, I awoke to sun and went to the window. The colour was even more vibrant than the day before. I smiled. My garden was a gift from dear friends, who knew that words alone weren't adequate to convey encouragement and hope. As spring slipped into summer and I moved from radiotherapy to chemo, this magnificent display greeted me daily. Tenderly nurtured and cared for by loved ones, my garden and I thrived and grew strong."
Jacqueline Hickey; diagnosed in 1993 at the age of 39; secretary, aspiring writer

They Really Want To

"Surround yourself with good people and let them do things for you. My neighbour came over to sit with me one day after my operation and was so insistent upon helping around the house that she washed an entire basket of clean clothes. We still laugh about that today."
Jennifer Wersal; diagnosed in 2000 at the age of 30; marketing executive

"A nurse friend came to stay with me for a week after my operation. I didn't actually need the physical help as much as someone to talk to. She had a little surprise gift every morning to get us started on a happy note."

Carol Hattler; diagnosed in 1999 at the age of 65; retired nurse

"If your friends want to take you to your treatments, accept their kind offer of help. They want to participate in your healing. Besides, it makes the trip more pleasant, and sometimes you are more exhausted than you realise."

Helen Wilker; diagnosed in 1999 at the age of 58; assistant teacher

"A simple thing such as a phone call to say 'Hello' or 'How are you?' means so much during treatment. A brief note saying 'Thinking of you' is never out of place."

Susan Clemente; diagnosed in 1990 at the age of 46; retired nurse

"My friends helped a lot. One of them rang me every day. I looked forward to our talks. Other friends sent me cards, flowers and food. It made me feel so good to know how much they cared."

Paula Porter; diagnosed in 2000 at the age of 47; telephone operator

"I had always cared for others and never allowed anyone to help me. After hearing my diagnosis, though, I didn't know how I was going to get through it. I learned during this time of surgery and treatments that I had to let go and allow others to help me. That was very hard for me to do. My best friend told me to practise doing it and it would get easier."

Carol Keen; diagnosed in 1999 at the age of 48; office clerk

"One of my dearest, oldest friends drove two hours in a snowstorm for just one night to help me blow-dry my hair . . . and my sister-in-law and husband took turns sleeping with me the first few nights, until we were all so tired that we woke up one morning, all three of us in bed!"

Bonnie Schneider; diagnosed in 1998 at the age of 45; audiologist

"When I came home from hospital, my best friend drove 700 miles to be there to take care of me. Did I feel special!"

E. Mary Lou Clauss; diagnosed in 1991 at the age of 55; retired nurse

"My best friend from school left her job and moved to my city to stay with me for the length of my treatments."
Asha Mevlana; diagnosed in 1999 at the age of 24; musician

"Accept help from others when offered, especially with meal preparation, childcare and lifts to medical appointments. It is not a sign of weakness. In fact, avoid thinking about how other people may judge you. You will be overwhelmed by the care and concern of others."
Mary Raffol; diagnosed in 1998 at the age of 44; teacher

"When I went into hospital for my operation, my friends got together and cleaned my house from top to bottom. When I came home from hospital, they brought me dinner every night for a week."
Carleen Muniz; diagnosed in 1998 at the age of 51; artist

"I concentrated on trying to hang in there and let my friends do the praying, and I truly believe it worked. I still get emotional when I think about how good everyone was to me."
Virginia Danczak; diagnosed in 1995 at the age of 58; phone company investigation centre

"One of my friends had breast cancer surgery and treatment exactly a year before my diagnosis. When I rang to tell her about my treatment plan, which included chemotherapy, she said, 'You can do this.' That simple – you can do this."
Faye Hardiman; diagnosed in 1998 at the age of 50; wife, mother, teacher

"Before my operation, each of my friends gave me the best of themselves in their individual ways. One told me to visualise his little finger and hold on to it as I went into the operating theatre. Another talked to the deer about me and flew a kite while thinking of me. A third one, knowing I do not embrace his religious beliefs, asked if I minded if he prayed for me. I am someone who gives from the heart for my friends. This was the first time when I have been the one who needed that heartfelt embrace. Remembering their loving gestures still brings tears to my eyes."
Jeanne Sturdevant; diagnosed in 1990 at the age of 45; artist

"It meant a lot to me to have someone take me to chemo treatments and keep me company. This often involved my husband or friends taking the day off work. One friend took me to a full-day chemo treatment when she was nine months pregnant and about to give birth! When neither my husband nor my friends could do it, I was driven by wonderful volunteers from a national cancer society. As an added bonus, those volunteers often have positive personal experiences to share."
Linda Perkins; diagnosed in 1999 at the age of 35; project manager

"Friends had special luncheons and parties for me. This was their way of showing me love and support. The radiotherapists even adjusted my time slot a couple of times when friends and I wanted to go out for lunch or a wine tasting."
Patti R. Martinez; diagnosed in 1999 at the age of 54; estate agent

"I wrote down the names of everyone who called offering to help, and then called them when I needed them. I threw a big thank-you party later (on my 50th birthday)!"
Judith Ormond; diagnosed in 1996 at the age of 49; symphony musician – piccolo

Goodies . . .

"One of the nicest things people can do for a cancer patient is to send food to the house, because it is so difficult and tiresome to have to cook. A meal sent in by caring friends tastes so much better!"
Susan Clemente; diagnosed in 1990 at the age of 46; retired nurse

"My friend Pat would ring or call and see me often. She would always ask, 'What can I do for you?' – not realising, I guess, that just phoning and coming to see me was more than enough. However, on one of her visits she brought dinner, cooked it, ate with me, and cleared away afterwards. It was just wonderful."
Carol Englund; diagnosed in 1994 at the age of 58; retired administrative assistant

"I have young children, and people brought over meals, instead of gifts. It was the most thoughtful thing that can be given to a woman

just back from major surgery. Friends also brought sweets for the kids."
Rhonda Sorrell; diagnosed in 1998 at the age of 43; special needs teacher

"Never take casseroles to families with teenagers. Take plain meat and potatoes, or, better still, order pizza and ice cream. A casserole will only make their dog fat!"
Mitzi Scarborough; diagnosed in 1999 at the age of 37; childminder

"Friends sent flowers and cards. I was bowled over by their thoughts, prayers and generosity. The most generous and most helpful gestures were made by the friends who either brought me dinner or took me out to dinner. They knew that I needed nourishment to fight the fatigue, and they were there for me."
Christine Foutris; diagnosed in 1999 at the age of 49; teacher

"The single most helpful thing was the delivery of meals which was organised by our church. Since we have no family in the area for support, the collective generosity of those women relieved me of having to think about preparing meals."
Wanda Null; diagnosed in 1986 at the age of 41; librarian

"A friend packed her car with frozen homemade soups and casseroles and drove 400 miles to help fill my freezer for those I-don't-feel-like-cooking days ahead. Another friend made a special effort to attend church that first Sunday after diagnosis, saying, 'I just didn't want you to sit by yourself today.' "
Betty Harris; diagnosed in 1999 at the age of 64; housewife

"Kathy, my incredible artist friend, hated cooking. So during her treatment, I took her out for her favourite Mexican food. She had two of the largest margaritas we'd ever seen, and we laughed through the entire meal!"
Sandra Baldwin Brown; friend of a survivor

"I got flowers, sweets, and presents, but the best thing was a gift voucher for a meal at my favourite restaurant."
Jill Gross; diagnosed in 2000 at the age of 51; head bank clerk

More Goodies . . .

"My daughter's 14th birthday was on the day I came home from hospital. My friend Diane met us at home with balloons, a home-made birthday cake and presents. This was Diane's gift to me."
Aileen Pandapas; diagnosed in 1989 at the age of 41; mother, volunteer, former secretary

"I had a wonderful support system. My colleagues sent food to my home, starting the day I came home from hospital and continuing for a couple of weeks. My best friends came and did work around the house, sat with me during my treatments, and took me out to lunch, shopping or the cinema."
Carol Keen; diagnosed in 1999 at the age of 48; office clerk

"The support that I received after diagnosis and surgery was beyond belief. I received more than 100 get well cards, and when I got home after my surgery, every night someone sent in dinner for my husband and me."
Jean Firkser; diagnosed in 1998 at the age of 66; housewife, retired receptionist

"Friends volunteered to drive me to appointments so that I never had to go anywhere alone. They volunteered to shop for groceries and even took out the rubbish regularly – down three flights of stairs!"
Carrie Drake; diagnosed in 1998 at the age of 42; administrative assistant

"A cleaner as a gift is really nice, even if only once."
Stephanie King; friend of two survivors

"A friend installed a detachable shower head, so I could wash my hair with all the bandages still on."
Judith Ormond; diagnosed in 1996 at the age of 49; symphony musician – piccolo

"Two gifts that meant a lot to me were very different: one was a pair of great-looking ear-rings for when I was better. The other was a small framed motto that says 'Tough times don't last. Tough people do.' I looked at it every day."
Suzanne Pollock; diagnosed in 1995 at the age of 50; stationer

"My book club friends kept dropping in with favourite books for me to read. They were the best medicine for sleeplessness, nausea or just spirit-lifting."
Betty Harris; diagnosed in 1999 at the age of 64; housewife

"When my friend Cathy was first diagnosed, I wrote her a short poem, since she loved poetry. Even when her treatment progressed, I continued to write and frame poems for her."
Nanette Thorsen-Snipes; friend of two survivors

"My friend's chemo treatments came during the summer and she bemoaned the fact that she could not enjoy all the fresh summer fruit she loved so much, as it was something she was told to avoid. So I found these terrific fruit gel candles in peach, strawberry, watermelon, honeydew and blueberry. I would light one for her as I read to her from some of her all-time favourite comfort books, like *Little Women* and *Anne of Green Gables*. The aroma was delicious and the next best thing to taking a bite. The house smelled like summer and put a smile on her face. It lifted her family's spirits as well. We are both avid readers and going back to the stories of her childhood was comforting to her. It transported her to another time and place, and helped pass the time. The sound of my voice, the familiar words and summer smells gave us some special moments together. We still buy these candles and light them whenever we sit down to read."
Cheryl Brinker; friend of Susan Thornton

"The most practical thing someone did for me was when my friend Linda came over and deadheaded my entire flower garden! She also sent me cards to celebrate the end of each chemo treatment."
Rosamary Amiet; diagnosed in 2000 at the age of 48; programme manager

"A friend brought me a little gift every Friday to celebrate the end of the week of radiotherapy. The last day of radiotherapy, my son came home from college to go with me. I took gifts to all of the radiotherapists."
Sharon Erbe; diagnosed in 1999 at the age of 54; nurse educator

More Goodies . . .

"I was overwhelmed by the number of cards, flowers and visitors I received. I never realised so many friends were thinking of me. I made new friends, too. The young nurses would gather in my room and talk about their pets and hobbies, as most were away from home. A waitress who worked in one of the restaurants where we frequently ate came to visit and brought the fried shrimp that she knew I loved. Another friend was away on holiday, but she rang up and sent cards every day."
Barbara C. Sumner; diagnosed in 1982 at the age of 59; housewife

"People's notes and gestures of support meant more than I could have imagined. Lesson learned – never pass up an opportunity to pick up the phone or send a card of encouragement. Better to make a mistake of commission than omission."
Patricia Baker; diagnosed in 1993 at the age of 49; housewife

"I received cards constantly. Some friends sent them weekly, and they often made me chuckle. Frequent 'just to let you know I'm thinking about you' phone calls kept my spirits way up. These things helped me know that I had not been forgotten and that no matter what I looked or felt like, my friends and family saw me as a valuable person."
Betty Harris; diagnosed in 1999 at the age of 64; housewife

"What helped me were the many, many cards and notes I received, especially from those who were also cancer survivors. Some of the people I had known quite well and I had never even known they had cancer. I certainly don't agree with keeping this hush-hush, as knowing others who have survived for a long time gave me a much brighter outlook on my future."
Sally Martel; diagnosed in 1996 at the age of 60; wife, mother, retired accountant

"I hung every single card I received on the wall in our living room. They reminded me of all those who loved me and cared about me. And I loved seeing my 'wall of cards' grow. I can't tell you how much it meant to me to know so many people were thinking about me and praying for me. It gave me strength and a daily boost.

When I finally took all my cards down, I felt my experience was over and done with."
Julie Crandall; diagnosed in 1998 at the age of 31; housewife and mother

"My role as a friend was just to be there. When my friends finished radiotherapy, I sent them both flowers to congratulate them on a job well done. I put on their cards that they were truly examples of courage to all of us."
Grace Trocco; friend of two survivors

"When my friend Susan was going through her chemotherapy, the three to four days after the treatments were the hardest for her. She often complained that the soles of her feet felt as though they were on fire. For those occasions, I found a wonderful lavender foot cream that I would put in the refrigerator at the start of my visit. Then the last thing I would do for her before I left was to get her all comfy in bed and give her a gentle foot massage with the cooled cream. I could almost immediately feel her body relax, and the lavender scent even helped her to relax enough to drift off, as sleep was also difficult for her at these times. To this day, we both continue to use this product."
Cheryl Brinker; friend of Susan Thornton

"When I was newly diagnosed, unbenown to me, a quilt friend put a notice in the local quilt e-mail directory asking people to make me a heart patch, a red heart on a white-on-white background, and write something on it. At that time, I didn't have a computer, so was not aware of what was happening and was rather confused when I started receiving these patches in the post! I spread them out on the dining-room table and every time I walked by, I got a wonderfully positive feeling from seeing the hearts and reading the messages. Then I extended the offer of participation to various non-quilting friends and family members. In the end, I had over a 100 patches, no two alike, and put together two quilts. They are not all red hearts on a white-on-white background – quilters tend to be somewhat independent! However, they all have a special place in my heart (pun intended), and I will always be thankful to those who gave of their hearts."
Sheilah Musselman; diagnosed in 1997 at the age of 56; nurse

Returning the Favour

"A colleague and friend who is also a breast cancer survivor gave me wise advice. She told me what I should ask my doctors, what I should wear and where I could buy what I needed. Every week for months she wrote me encouraging notes. 'Courage is fear with prayer' was my very favourite. When I asked how I could ever thank her enough, she answered that I should do for others what she'd done for me. At the time I had hoped to be spared that, but two of my colleagues at school this year needed advice, and I was glad and proud to help them."
Christine Foutris; diagnosed in 1999 at the age of 49; teacher

"One of the most helpful things people in my neighbourhood did was prepare meals for our family. Twenty-five women from my small community signed up to do it five days a week for six months!! It was wonderful, and I got visitors every day. Now, I have the opportunity to give back to another friend in our community who has recently been diagnosed. It's great being on the receiving end, but I think the giving makes you feel even better."
Anita Leuzzi; diagnosed in 1997 at the age of 45; legal secretary

"Promise yourself that you will return the kindnesses that were offered to you. One day it will be your turn to help, and you will feel good about reciprocating."
Mary Raffol; diagnosed in 1998 at the age of 44; teacher

"Friends are more important to me since my operation. It takes time to have friends, time and effort that we don't always have when we're looking after our families or working. But my priorities have changed."
Anne Jacobs; diagnosed in 1999 at the age of 62; managing partner, estate agency

"When I went in for a mammogram, I saw a friend, Kim, sitting there. I talked to her and found that my experience had prompted her to get a mammogram."
Sandy Williams; diagnosed in 1999 at the age of 51; children's public librarian

9 · The Workplace

Making It User-Friendly

There's nothing like being your own boss. In that sense, I had the best possible scenario when it came to working through breast cancer treatment. Yes, I work to a deadline, but the deadline that I set for myself is usually a month or more before the one that my publisher sets for me. This means I have leeway should something crop up. It certainly took the pressure off when I was diagnosed.

Another good thing about being your own boss is being able to work at home. I wore tracksuits. I wore big men's shirts. I sat with a hotwater bottle between the chair and my back (no one *told* me my back would hurt when my chest wall was pushed out to make room for new breasts – but that does get better, ladies), and no one gave me strange looks. I didn't have to apologise or explain when I took off for a couple of hours to have radiotherapy or a nap.

Not everyone has this luxury. Occupation-wise, *UPLIFT* survivors range from bus driver to musician to banker. We have dentists and dental nurses, lawyers and legal assistants, microbiologists, psychotherapists and midwives. We have a journalist. We have architects, sales clerks and telephone operators. We have a symphony musician.

If I were to single out the occupation with the heaviest concentration of submitters, it would be teachers – but then, teachers do like to write. There are also a striking number of nurses in the group. Of course, they were in a prime position to learn about this project and care about passing on their advice. Lord knows, they've seen the downside of women who are in the dark.

And there were wives and mums galore – far more than are listed in the credits – and I'm sorry for that. When people were asked about their occupation, they often listed their outside-the-home job, when the content of their submissions clearly suggests that they juggle inside-the-home jobs as well.

Inside or outside, an amazing number of women said that they worked right through their treatment. I can identify with these women. For me, work was an escape. It enabled me to minimise the impact of having breast cancer and was a reminder that life went on.

Not every woman works right through, and remarks from these women are included here, too. They'll tell you about the flexibility of their bosses and about how taking time off worked for them.

Worked for them. That's the key, here. What works for one woman may not work for another. What works in one job may not work in another. The thing is, you need to take a step back, think about yourself and your situation, then speak up about what may work for you. In every situation, you have choices, and the choices are all good. What pleases one woman may not please another.

Which is why they have menus in restaurants, as my dad used to say.

Spilling the Beans

"I never made a secret of my diagnosis. My staff knew almost as soon as my family. I did try to choose carefully the time and circumstances when I told friends and acquaintances – I did not want to appear melodramatic, but I also didn't want people to find out from a source other than me. I felt strongly that I was the best source of information about my illness, and I knew I felt good and looked good."

Wanda Null; diagnosed in 1986 at the age of 41; librarian

"Talking about my diagnosis, my appointments, my procedures and my observations was one of the best things I could have done. By sharing my experiences, I was able to reduce some of the fear

that my friends, family, colleagues and I were experiencing. Everyone at work has been supportive. I really believe that because I was open and honest, I was able to educate them. When people become educated about a subject, they become less fearful of it. I encourage everyone to ask whatever questions they might have."
Val Long; diagnosed in 1999 at the age of 47; administrative assistant

"I am a hairdresser, so I can make my own schedule, with chemo and all. Losing my hair was the worst, but I bought a wig that looked like my own hair, so no one really knew. Customers of the salon who have heard I have cancer have come to me telling of their stories with the disease. I've found support everywhere!"
Sharon Daniels; diagnosed in 2000 at the age of 49; hairdresser, wig shop owner

"How did I do it (juggle breast cancer and work)? I adopted a slight variation of the notorious 'don't ask, don't tell' policy. On the private side, only a few close friends and family members heard the news about my breast cancer diagnosis. On the professional side, I did not share details about my health crisis with anyone outside my organisation. When customers made comments (once I was wearing a wig), like 'Oh, you've changed your hair!' I responded with a simple, 'Yes, I have.' I acknowledged. I smiled. Nothing more. Good thing nobody asked, 'Hey, where are your eyebrows and eyelashes?' With practice, simple responses that revealed nothing became automatic. This worked for me; I could maintain my privacy and productivity level during treatment. I didn't have to drain my energies dealing with everyone else's level of discomfort with cancer. But most importantly, I could stay focused on work and address critical health issues at the same time."
Alysa Cummings; diagnosed in 1998 at the age of 45; educational trainer

"I discovered my cancer three weeks before the opening night of my favourite musical, *A Funny Thing Happened on the Way to the Forum*. The stress of that, plus a four-week cold, took its toll. I looked terrible. Fellow teachers asked me if my cough was going to kill me. Frightened that they were right, I would run away to cry. A simple 'How are you?' seemed inane; I wanted to answer 'I'm afraid I'm going to die from cancer. How are you?' I had always stressed honesty with my pupils, but I was not composed enough to tell them anything. Fearing what a crisis might do to a secondary school cast, and thinking this would be the last show I ever directed, I decided to enjoy Saturday's closing night and go in for surgery the following Monday. I also decided to write a letter to the students, and my musical director generously agreed to read it to them. In the letter, I stated the situation, my planned procedures, and my doctor's optimism for my total recovery. I reminded my pupils of their many resources, appealing to their sense of creativity in solving artistic and personal problems. I ended my letter with 'When I return, we will learn and produce art together.' Almost a decade later, I still communicate with many of these pupils, and we're all still learning and producing art."

Judy Thibault Klevins; diagnosed in 1992 at the age of 47; arts teacher

"My most difficult task was telling my middle-school pupils that I had breast cancer. I would be absent for the remainder of the term, and I felt that they had a right to know why. I came to school on what was to be my last day, and had decided to tell the pupils straight after morning assembly. I hadn't a clue what I would say or how they would receive the news. Would they be glad I was leaving? Would the boys snigger at my condition? I don't exactly remember what I said, but I gave them the facts – that I had breast cancer, that I would need an operation, and that I was scared. I told them that they were approaching the best time of the academic year – the latter part of the spring term – and that I would miss sharing it with them. I'm not sure what else I said, but when I really looked at my kids, I was astonished to see crying, upset children. My classes that day began in a sombre fashion, but we discussed my condition and they shared stories about cancer in their own families, and they each hugged me as they left the classroom. I had an Arab pupil at the time who told me that he had never before prayed for a Christian, but he promised to pray for me. I think that being a teacher is special, but during a time of crisis, pupils can be your best ally. After the assembly, the teachers were greeted by crying kids entering their classrooms. It ended up being a school-wide occasion. All the faculty were helpful in discussing the problem of breast cancer, the librarian made books available, the head of the Science Department made materials available to all of his classes. By 9 o'clock the flowers started arriving in my classroom – my pupils and their parents were sending them. I was amazed that many of the boys, in particular, called their mothers to give them the news. At one point, the headmaster called me in to tell me that my pupils were sneaking off to the local flower shop and that he was going to let them continue to do so. The kids were so wonderful that I left school elated. Shortly after I arrived home, my surgeon called to inform me that the 'just in case' biopsy of my other breast showed cancer, and that I would need surgery on both breasts. My mood at that time had been so positively influenced by my pupils that I barely reacted. I took the news calmly and told her of my day. Although the day of surgery was one of the scariest days of my life, the experience with my pupils helped me face it with confidence."

Lee Williams; diagnosed in 1996 at the age of 56; teacher

A Workplace Manual

"Here are the strategies that helped me maintain that crucial balance between cancer and work: (1) I scheduled doctor's appointments early in the day or at the beginning of their surgeries. This way I was in and out of the surgery nice and fast. Doctors' schedules seem to back up as the day wears on. (2) Since radiotherapy treatments are scheduled daily at the same time for six weeks, I begged and grovelled to get a time slot near the end of the business day. (3) I planned my operations (especially the elective reconstruction procedures) for Fridays, holidays, or slow times for business. Weekends are great times to recuperate and get back on your feet without losing precious work time or taking days off sick. (4) I got an understudy and trained her. When I knew that I would not be feeling my best, (i.e., the first three days after a chemo infusion), I arranged the understudy to work side by side with me. That way I had a safety net."

Alysa Cummings; diagnosed in 1998 at the age of 45; educational trainer

"My young pupils cherished me and took care of me. They wouldn't let me lift or carry anything because they knew I wasn't supposed to be using my arm at that time."

Sue Watson; diagnosed in 1996 at the age of 53; teacher

"While I was having treatments, I worked every day, but I finally realised that it was okay to have naps. Once I figured this out, it

helped me get through a hard week a little better. My body let me know what it needed."
Michele Marks; diagnosed in 1996 at the age of 33; CAD operator

"My boss got me a laptop so that I could work from home on the days I didn't feel well."
Asha Mevlana; diagnosed in 1999 at the age of 24; musician

"My boss at the time was my brother. He suggested I go for radio-therapy in the morning, work a few hours, then go home and rest in the afternoons. That is what I did, because even though I looked great, I was unbelievably tired. When illness comes, we need to listen to our bodies and give them the time to rest and recover. I hadn't anticipated it, but those afternoon hours became a truly peaceful, nurturing time to read and rest and enjoy peace and quiet."
Deb Haney; diagnosed in 1996 at the age of 48; administrative assistant, artist

"I work at a secondary school with over 1,200 pupils. During chemo, I was concerned about being exposed to so many people and possibly falling ill. The school authorities were great. They purchased a telephone headset for me to use, so that I wouldn't be exposed to unnecessary germs."
Linda Jones Burns; diagnosed in 2000 at the age of 40; school registrar

"In the workplace, it was helpful when people stayed away from me when they had colds. The owner of the company told me to work only when I was up to it, and my bosses were patient with my distraction and my distracting others. There were lots of questions, and I answered them all. I wanted to educate everybody along with myself. Work was my salvation. My fellow employees were supportive and continue to be so in my efforts to raise funds for cancer research. On the flip side, I've become the company support person on breast health. I even had my surgeon come and give a talk."
Deborah J. P. Schur; diagnosed in 1994 at the age of 43; sales rep

"It was very important to me to show people that I was alive and well. I rested between patients at the office, had a light schedule, and didn't do housework. I saved my energy for the office. My

husband accompanied me to many functions and meetings at our children's school. We would never stay long, but I wanted to show my face."
A survivor; diagnosed in 1998 at the age of 45; dentist

"I juggled cancer and work by just giving up some things, like housework. I discovered that the house could go for weeks without being vacuumed or dusted – and not only did the sky not fall, it didn't even crack!"
Rosamary Amiet; diagnosed in 2000 at the age of 48; programme manager

"If you are a large-breasted woman who has a lumpectomy with radiotherapy, and you're working during treatment, you face a dilemma. You don't want to go without a bra in the workplace, because you feel like a cow! You can't wear a bra with bones or underwires, because they put pressure on the affected area. You need wide straps so that nothing digs into your shoulders, and you need a fabric that doesn't irritate your skin. During radiotherapy, sexy goes out of the door, and comfort is the watchword! A full-figure comfortable bra fit the bill for me. Go to a shop that has a professional fitter and try on everything. I'd suggest buying one of the most comfortable bras and trying it out for a week before buying another one. The bra can be washed out every night. That way you haven't wasted a fortune on bras, only to find that they don't go the distance."
Sharon Irons Strempski; diagnosed in 1997 at the age of 52; nurse

"The company I work for was very supportive, giving me time off when needed and consoling me when I felt down. I was on disability pay for a few months and then returned to work while still getting chemo treatments."
Sandy Mark; diagnosed in 1998 at the age of 55; administrative assistant

Better than a Christmas Bonus

"I always knew I enjoyed the people I work with. But I never knew that they loved me, that they would be there for me, that they would cheer me up, encourage me, make me laugh, that they

would help me believe in myself, so that I would know that I'd get well!"
Carolyn Stein; diagnosed in 1998 at the age of 45; medical secretary

"The people I work with brought a meal for every night of the week for three weeks, so that my family didn't have to worry about any of it. These colleagues all gave days of sick leave to me so that I would not have to go a day without pay. I only missed work when I absolutely had to. If I sat around doing nothing, I felt worse! The best thing I did was go to work and walk . . . walk . . . walk."
Pam Waddell; diagnosed in 1998 at the age of 38; writer, teacher's assistant

"I missed work for my operation and the six weeks after it. My boss brought a baked Alaska to the hospital as a gift. We had no knife or plates, but the nurses loved it. Later he brought work to my house for me."
Irene Louise; diagnosed in 1995 at the age of 41; retired PA

"I worked with some of the best people. They called to check up on me. One friend went to all of my appointments with me. The supervisors kept telling me not to worry about the time off, and they kept paying me."
Michele Marks; diagnosed in 1996 at the age of 33; CAD operator

"My colleagues organised a rota whereby someone brought me home-cooked food at least once a week. A quiche or casserole lasted several days!"
Carrie Drake; diagnosed in 1998 at the age of 42; administrative assistant

"When I was first diagnosed, I was worried about losing my job. But everyone at work was very caring. They were always asking for updates on my progress. A colleague offered to shave my head in stages so that it would not be so devastating all at once. We would cut a little each week until it was time to shave it all."
Kathy Rabassa; diagnosed in 1999 at the age of 34; administrative assistant

"My operation was in the summer holidays, and I resumed work the following autumn. During this time, I underwent chemotherapy

and radiotherapy. My colleagues did many small things to make my life easier. They formed a dinner 'brigade' and took turns making dinner for us on my 'ill from chemo' days. They were aware that I would have temporary memory loss because of the drugs, so instead of just telling me about a problem with a certain child, they would write me 'love' notes and put them on my office door to gently remind me. My headmistress allowed me to take my usual lunch break to have radiotherapy. When this took longer than the allotted time, she reasoned that I had spent many breaks working with teachers or children, and had earned at least that much time to use for this purpose. Therefore, I didn't lose work time for those appointments. It was so important for me to be 'normal' and these men and women provided me with that."
Brenda Carr; diagnosed in 1988 at the age of 40; wife, mother, retired school counsellor

"I work with a wonderful group of people. After learning of my breast cancer, I received gifts almost daily. This was better than Christmas or my birthday! The day before my operation, they surprised me with breakfast . . . a going-away party for my breast!"
Rosamary Amiet; diagnosed in 2000 at the age of 48; programme manager

"I had not been at my job a year, so I had not accumulated much holiday. The people there donated their sick leave and holidays to me to use for the bad days during chemo, and for my operation and recovery. Their kindness will always be appreciated and remembered."
Gwen Loverink; diagnosed in 1994 at the age of 34; police dispatcher

"I was blessed to work in an educational authority personnel department with colleagues who were incredibly supportive and understanding. Every day for six weeks, I joked that I was actually going to the beach to work on my tan, rather than heading to hospital for my daily dose of rays. On the morning of my last treatment, I took in a 'beach picnic' for my 'office family'. We had bagels in a bucket, cream cheese on a spade, and cool fruit juice from the blender, and I gave everyone a bright Hawaiian lei. In turn, they surprised me with a beautiful Estée Lauder heart-shaped compact. Later I engraved on it the words 'Beach Party, December

3, 1999'. It is a constant reminder to me of the love and support of very dear friends."
Paula Linman; diagnosed in 1999 at the age of 48; educational authority personnel secretary

"Since I had taken time off work to focus on and get through treatments, that meant my husband had to work more. My friends were worried that I was not having enough fun, so we would often meet for lunch. They would always pick up the tab, knowing that my husband and I were counting every penny. One Sunday, my friends rang to say that they were coming to babysit for my two boys and that they were ordering my husband and me out for a meal. When they arrived, they handed my husband a gift voucher for the most romantic restaurant. Off we went and enjoyed a most delicious dinner. Later, when I entered my bedroom, I noticed a single rose on our pillows. Under the rose was a card, with good wishes from all the people I worked with. Enclosed was a cheque. The card said that the money was to be used for whatever I felt my family needed it for. While a trip to Disneyworld sounded very appealing, the bills were mounting up. This gift allowed us to make two mortgage payments. It is a true friend who goes the extra mile to find what it is that you and your family really need."
Cindy Fiedler; diagnosed in 1998 at the age of 40; nurse, mother

"I was stunned by the love and support I received from friends and colleagues during my illness. When I returned to work, I wrote this Top Ten list and read it at a department gathering.

Top Ten Reasons Why Having Cancer Is Not *Completely Horrible*

No. 10 I lost ten pounds.
No. 9 I read several books.
No. 8 I got lots of e-mails, cards and presents.
No. 7 I had eight months off with disability income.
No. 6 I saved a lot of money on haircuts and shampoo.
No. 5 I learned to appreciate nose hair.
No. 4 I could watch daytime TV.
No. 3 I met strong, inspiring women.

No.   2 My husband and I are even closer.
And the No. 1 reason why having cancer is not completely horrible
is . . . that the people who love me have told me so."
Lisette; diagnosed in 1999 at the age of 47; business analyst

Keep On Truckin'

"I had just qualified as a lawyer when I was diagnosed. Work was my
salvation. I went back to it ten weeks after my mastectomy and only
remember missing two days during my six months of chemo."
Barbara Jentis; diagnosed in 1983 at the age of 41; lawyer

"Thank goodness for children. I have a group that comes before
the library opens to the public. They are bright and alert. As I do
their story time I lose myself in their expressions and responses."
Sandy Williams; diagnosed in 1999 at the age of 51; children's public
librarian

"I was told by the people at work to take all the time I needed. But
I didn't miss work. Keeping busy was my salvation. Each day, I put
on make-up and a smile. When my hair fell out, I put on a great
wig. It cost a fortune, but it was money well spent. No one knew it
was not my hair."
Frances Gallello; diagnosed in 2000 at the age of 51; mental health
assistant

"I worked through the whole thing. I think that my breast cancer
bothered others more than it bothered me."
Carleen Muniz; diagnosed in 1998 at the age of 51; artist

"I learned to do things differently at work as a school bus driver to
help take the pressure off just one arm."
Mary Ann Budnick; diagnosed in 1991 at the age of 44; school bus driver

"When my sister was diagnosed with breast cancer, I thought it
would only strike one sister. Boy, was I wrong. Three years later, I
was diagnosed, and had a lumpectomy, chemotherapy and six
weeks of radiotherapy. I've been selling houses on commission for
22 years – I'm divorced and support myself – so having to go into
hospital wasn't exactly what I wanted. The good news is, I spent two

days at home resting, then I went out and sold two houses with one side of my chest bound and aching!"
Patti R. Martinez; diagnosed in 1999 at the age of 54; estate agent

"I worked with 20 women at the office. They were loving, caring and devoted to me, and my boss was extremely generous and giving. Work helped to bridge the gap for me, and I resumed as much of my lifestyle as I could without any alterations."
Alyce Feinstein; diagnosed in 1993 at the age of 58; administrative assistant

"Stay busy. I was fortunate to work for a bank that allowed me to work flexible hours."
Jill Gross; diagnosed in 2000 at the age of 51; head bank clerk

"The only work I missed was during my surgery. I worked every day while I went through chemo, even though I was tired. It made me feel as though there was some semblance of normality in my life."
Barbara Moro; diagnosed in 1999 at the age of 57; law secretary

After the Storm

"I went to work every day and had a smile for everyone. I still do. When you smile, everyone around you knows you're okay."
Pam Waddell; diagnosed in 1998 at the age of 38; writer, teacher's assistant

"I felt feminine once I had my new prosthesis, as I had lost a stone and wore a new dress on my return to work. I felt they would all look and think, 'Which side was it?' However, when they saw me, they were so glad, they hugged me and kissed me, and we all laughed. I felt good from then on."
Irene Louise; diagnosed in 1995 at the age of 41; retired executive secretary

"I sent out a company-wide e-mail where I work, urging younger female employees to have mammograms and examine themselves regularly. Twelve women in my office arranged mammograms that week. The company now plans to have a mobile mammogram unit in the car park."
Joy West; diagnosed in 2000 at the age of 34; advertising account co-ordinator

"How did I juggle breast cancer and work? I was determined to maintain an appearance of normality as I organised operations, chemotherapy, radiotherapy and doctor's appointments while running a small business. Two years after diagnosis, I am pleased to report that my business is thriving, and (touch wood) according to my oncologist, so am I."

Alysa Cummings; diagnosed in 1998 at the age of 45; educational trainer

10 Support Groups

From Traditional to Offbeat

"A breast cancer diagnosis puts you into an exclusive club. You wouldn't choose to join it, but once you do, you find a sisterhood like no other." This thought was sent in by Stephanie King, an oncology nurse who passed it along second-hand, but the sentiment was too good not to pass it on again. Indeed, one of the most meaningful parts of my experience with this book has been meeting survivors. Yes, there's an instant rapport. Regardless of how old we are, where we live or what treatment choices we made, having gone through breast cancer gives us a connection. Never having joined a support group, I'm experiencing this bond for the very first time.

Why didn't I join a support group? There are several reasons, not the least of which had to do with time. Between family, career and cancer treatment, I was busy enough; attending a weekly support group meeting would have been one commitment too many. There was also the privacy issue; even back then, my name was recognisable, and I was trying to keep word of my cancer quiet. I was also afraid of joining a support group, because there was a chance that someone in the group might die, and I didn't think I could handle that.

No, a traditional support group didn't appeal to me, but, looking back, I would have liked to have had a 'cancer buddy'. I did try once. On a recommendation, I phoned the friend of a friend, but the woman so depressed me that I put the phone down and cried. She was clearly the wrong person for me, not upbeat at all. But many survivors have found the right person, and the experience sounds wonderful.

For the purposes of this chapter, I use the term 'group' in its loosest form. There can be a 'group' of 30, a 'group' of eight or a 'group' of two. Indeed, in the course of organising *UPLIFT*, I learned about many different sizes of groups. I've organised this chapter along those lines. There are traditional support groups that meet at regular times, often in a hospital setting. Some are defined by age, some by the time from diagnosis. There are support pairings – some set up by a hospital, some by a friend, some by a fluke. There are *unusual* support vehicles, one of the most promising being cyberspace.

And then, of course, there's *UPLIFT*. It is definitely a support group and just the kind that would have worked for me. I could have availed myself of it from the privacy of my bedroom, could have spent five minutes with it or an hour, could have picked up bits of advice and got the encouragement that I wanted, could have been absolutely, positively assured of an optimistic response from hundreds of women. In the course of compiling this book, I corresponded with many of its contributors. We shared theories and compared stories to the extent that I do now consider them friends. So here is another kind of support group. If I had to fit *UPLIFT* into one of the slots in this chapter, it would be "Off the Beaten Path".

Of course you can have *UPLIFT* and another support group, too! Remember, though, what works for one woman may not work for another. As in so many other aspects of breast cancer survival, there are choices. Here are the different kinds of support groups. Pick yours.

Tried and True

"A friend of mine was going through her illness at the same time as I was. I wanted to be supportive of her, so I went with her to a support group at a local hospital. I found that I benefited greatly from attending those meetings. I highly recommend support groups for a better recovery result. Talking to others who are going through the same ordeal can be very comforting. Not only do you help

yourself, but it makes you feel better when you can help others as well."
Sheila Steinhauser; diagnosed in 1985 at the age of 41; office manager

"My support group filled in the cracks when I needed it most. We shared everything together and learned from one another. There was a common bond. I met many women during this period, and we held nothing back."
Alyce Feinstein; diagnosed in 1993 at the age of 58; administrative assistant

"One of the best pieces of advice I can give is to have someone to talk to – a support group to pick up on the things that you can't do – someone to just hang out with, to lean on."
Michele Marks; diagnosed in 1996 at the age of 33; CAD operator

"Consider joining a local support group even though it may not be your thing. That way, you will always have somewhere to talk things over in the company of people who understand."
Mary Raffol; diagnosed in 1998 at the age of 44; teacher

"Get into a support group as soon as you're diagnosed. I got into mine late, which I regret. The place I go has three levels – newly diagnosed and in treatment, after treatment, and three or more years after treatment."
Sharon Irons Strempski; diagnosed in 1997 at the age of 52; nurse

"My women's group is a tool all cancer patients need to have."
Nan Comstock; diagnosed in 1988 at the age of 39; self-employed

"Through my support group, I'm regaining the power that cancer has taken from me. I can now say without reservation, 'God never closes a door without opening a window, and the view from the window he's opened is beautiful.'"
Joy West; diagnosed in 2000 at the age of 34; advertising account co-ordinator

"The breast cancer survivors of my support group were my dearest support. My time with them has helped me reach the place in my life where I can say that breast cancer has been a gift. It has

changed my life. It took me a while to get to this point, though. In the beginning, when I was in pain, one of the support group facilitators, a breast cancer survivor herself, said that I should feel the pain like a thunderstorm – that it is there and then will pass."
Bonnie Schneider; diagnosed in 1998 at the age of 45; audiologist

"I had family members coming and helping out around the house, and friends bringing meals. At first I felt upset that they were all doing this stuff for me, but by the end of my first four cycles of chemo, I was worn out and knew I needed help. When I got discouraged and fearful, I talked to a nurse. That helped. I also joined a support group. Even though the women were older than me (I was 24), we all had breast cancer in common. They have been a wonderful support for me."
Candice Jaeger; diagnosed in 2000 at the age of 24; wife and mother

"I have learned that we do not have to face this alone. Yes, our families are a tremendous support, but it is important to share our feelings with others who know exactly how we feel – and they also know how to help our family members deal with it too."
Rose Marie Clark; diagnosed in 1996 at the age of 50; retired

"I started my own cancer support with women in my area, and I have learned to basically use my cancer as a tool for spiritual awakening. I became a Reiki Master last year. Reiki is a form of energy healing and I have a nursing background. I have begun a small practice helping to teach men and women how to use their experience with cancer as their tool for growth by tapping into their inherent wisdom. It is too easy to let the fear and uncertainty that comes with getting cancer take control."
Sandy Rodgers; diagnosed in 1999 at the age of 44; housewife, mother, nurse, Reiki Master

"Four months after my operation, I looked for a support group. I felt that I needed to be with other women who had been there, so that I could gather some strength and get a better balance in my life. It was a great thing to do. The group was lively and friendly. Newcomers got to meet women who'd had similar surgery. Questions were answered and fears were understood. No one really knows how you're feeling unless they have been there too. The truth is, cancer has made my life richer. I never thought I would say that, but it has. I now volunteer in a cancer resource library and help others find information about their disease."

Pauline Hughes; diagnosed in 1997 at the age of 61; retired nurse

One Other Person

"The hospital set me up with a 'buddy' who was going through similar treatment and who was around the same age as me. She became one of my best friends during this time. She understood everything about the sickness and anxiety that I didn't want to pile on my friends. It was critical to have someone who really understood what I was going through."

Asha Mevlana; diagnosed in 1999 at the age of 24; musician

"I met a wonderful woman while we were both undergoing radiotherapy. She had a great face and hat, so I asked where she got the hat, and we chatted for hours. She has become a very dear friend. She and I feel a kinship that only cancer survivors know. I did find out where she got the hat and have since recommended them to many people."

Susan Clemente; diagnosed in 1990 at the age of 46; retired nurse

"One of the best things that can happen? Someone answered my e-mail request for information when I couldn't find literature. She became my mentor, giving me questions to ask and explaining what I might have missed."

Anne Jacobs; diagnosed in 1999 at the age of 62; managing partner, estate agency

"Six weeks after getting married, I was diagnosed with breast cancer. I was 27. My diagnosis came as a shock to everyone! My former college friend's mother, a breast cancer survivor herself, rang me and recommended a book that helped me understand the diagnosis and prepare questions for my doctors."

Beth Compton; diagnosed in 1995 at the age of 27; civil engineer

"I believe that developing a positive comradery with a person who has walked in your shoes can be very helpful and encouraging."

Becky Honeycutt; diagnosed in 1995 at the age of 53; nurse

"Get to know some women who are survivors – they are not hard to find! Talking to women who have been survivors for five years, 14 years, or 39-plus years encourages me. I think of these women's stories when my own fears surface."
Faye Hardiman; diagnosed in 1998 at the age of 50; wife, mother, teacher

"Find someone who has been down this path to be your mentor! My priest's wife's cousin Alma was sent by God. Although it was less than two years since her own diagnosis, she was a tremendous support. We e-mailed and talked on the phone. She told me to ask for tests that would not have been done had I not asked. My husband, Wally, said that it was a big emotional relief for him to know that I had a 'lay expert' I could turn to at any point."
Monica May; diagnosed in 1997 at the age of 40; consultant

"As soon as I was diagnosed, a volunteer came and spent the day with me. She was wonderful! We laughed, cried and ate junk food. I felt much better by the time she left. She had survived, and I could too."
Mitzi Scarborough; diagnosed in 1999 at the age of 37; childminder

"Many people, a lot of them strangers, took the time to tell me of their own cancer battle and survival. I hadn't even known they'd had cancer. Their stories encouraged me and gave me hope. I try to do the same for others."
Sue Watson; diagnosed in 1996 at the age of 53; teacher

"I am a medical social worker. I might have got helpful advice from my colleagues, but I was not comfortable sharing my diagnosis with them for fear of being treated differently by patients and staff. So the most help and excellent advice came from the friend of a friend, whom to this day I have never met. Barbara, who is also a survivor, remained a voice on the telephone who helped me work through treatment choices and gave wonderful advice as to how to negotiate the next few months of my life. She said that it was okay not to wear a bra if I wasn't comfortable with it during the weeks of radiotherapy, that it was okay to disagree with my doctor (I changed doctors before radiotherapy began), that it was okay to cry and lean on my spouse, and that I do not have to know every-

thing. She said that this time I was allowed to be the patient. I was the one in charge of my life decisions. She helped me to see that I needed to set my coping goals for one minute at a time, one hour at a time, one day at a time – and then to realise, yes, I can do this!"
Nancie Watson; diagnosed in 1995 at the age of 50; social worker

"I recommend going to your treatments alone. You're bound to meet and talk to your fellow chemo and/or radiotherapy patients. It's almost like a support group. If you have a family member or friend with you, you are less likely to talk to anyone else. Also, going by yourself makes it seem more like just another doctor's appointment, rather than a big ordeal. I got really friendly with a couple of my oncology nurses. They were wonderful . . . and very funny! Sometimes I'd leave there thinking 'How in the world did I have fun at a chemo treatment?' Not that I wasn't *very* happy when I had my *last* treatment!"
Deborah Lambert; diagnosed in 2000 at the age of 47; medical secretary

"In the paper, I read a letter about a 'must have' booklet for cancer patients. I rang up and ordered one. The last question they asked me was, 'Would you like a cancer survivor to ring you?' '*No! I would not!*' I thought, but instead, the single word 'Yes' came out.

"For several weeks, I cried and cried. One particularly bad night, the phone rang. I picked it up. A woman said that her name was Connie and asked whether I had time to chat. 'Yes,' I whispered, and she asked how I was doing. 'Not so good,' I said. 'I can't stop crying. When will I stop crying and feeling sorry for myself?' Connie said, 'One day, it will just stop. You'll be okay. We all need time to mourn, time to be sad, and it's okay to cry.' She went on to tell me that she cried a lot at first. She gave all her clothes away except a dress, a skirt and a blouse. Days, weeks, months went by. She didn't die, but she had no clothes! That was 20 years ago. That night, I began to heal – laughing for the first time in a long, long time. That night, I learned tears are okay. Tears are a part of healing."
Jinny Morrison; diagnosed in 1998 at the age of 55; bus assistant for mentally retarded adults

Off the Beaten Path

"I found conventional support group meetings difficult, so I

formed my own support dinner group. We would dine out every couple of months to discuss having breast cancer. We also shared stories of our spouses, children and travels."
Deborah J. P. Schur; diagnosed in 1994 at the age of 43; sales rep

"When they found cancer in one breast, I decided on a prophylactic mastectomy of the other. Afterwards, I formed what I tenderly call the 'Double or Nothing Club' for all my friends who have had bilateral mastectomies."
Aileen Pandapas; diagnosed in 1989 at the age of 41; mother, volunteer, former secretary

"The most practical thing I did after diagnosis was to start a support group for breast cancer survivors in their twenties and thirties. We call ourselves the 'Big C Chicks' and now number around 15 members. Our mission is not only to support and mentor one another, but to educate our peers that no one is too young to have breast cancer."
Joy West; diagnosed in 2000 at the age of 34; advertising account co-ordinator

"We have a large family, and my brother and sister-in-law have a very large circle of friends and business associates. When my sister-in-law was in hospital, the process of keeping everyone updated was daunting. So my brother set up a website devoted to his wife's health and recovery status. He entered information every day, and visitors to the site were encouraged to sign the guest book, which was a way to send an e-mail to my sister-in-law or brother. It was a fantastic way to keep everyone updated and served as a way for all of us to schedule visits, plus my sister-in-law got to see how many people were out there rooting for her."
Wendy Page; sister-in-law of Barbra Marcus Kolton

"I didn't want to go to the vicar's 40th birthday party, but my husband insisted that we go for a while. We were met by many familiar faces, helium balloons, food, cake, drinks and loving hugs. Two friends, each of whom had been free of breast cancer for more than 20 years, shared stories with me. Another friend, who had recently finished chemo, assured me that if I had to have it, the doctors would give me medicine to keep me from

getting so terribly sick. My spirits rose. I felt positive again. I could do this."
Sandy Williams; diagnosed in 1999 at the age of 51; children's public librarian

" 'There is no such thing as a problem without a gift for you in its hands.' One of the gifts I received came in the form of a four-day retreat with a national cancer foundation. I was with ten other women who'd had breast cancer. We talked, laughed and sometimes cried together. We went kayaking and I recall seeing trees hanging from cliffs with their roots totally exposed. I commented to the other woman in my kayak, 'Trees aren't supposed to live like that, with their roots all exposed to the elements, hanging from the edge of a cliff. But the will to survive is strong, and we, too, can continue to thrive with less than optimal conditions, just like those trees.' One of the women at this retreat was a petite grey-haired woman, probably in her sixties, who had been blind from birth and had two glass eyes. Our first night, she got up and sang – a rap song no less – about her wahddy dahddy do, which was the name she had come up with for the flap of skin under your armpit after a mastectomy. She had us all just roaring with laughter. She went kayaking for the first time in her life on this retreat."
Gracie Schwingel; diagnosed in 1998 at the age of 51; secretary

"When I was diagnosed with breast cancer, I e-mailed a few friends to let them know. One friend who was not on the list e-mailed me to say, 'We're your friends in the bad times as well as the good!' As a result, I wrote to two lists of friends, whom I dubbed 'Supergals' and 'Power Pals'. I gave them permission to pass on my e-mail to anyone they felt it would help. The list grew over the next six months from 14 to over 200. I sent 'Updates from Deb' periodically to describe what I was going through so they could understand the tests and procedures. Six months later, I'd received over 1,300 e-mail messages back. Two of my favourites were 'Because of your updates and courage, my mum went to have a mammogram for the first time in four years!' and 'My mum has breast cancer, too, and is about three weeks behind you in treatment – I've been forwarding your updates and she is no longer afraid, because she knows what to expect.' I've realised that breast cancer was a blessing, not a curse. Discovering that people truly

care about me was wonderful. Being able to help others going through something similar was awesome."
Deb Haggerty; diagnosed in 1999 at the age of 51; professional speaker

"A unique experience I had with breast cancer was that I 'met' a woman online who was diagnosed at the same time I was. She and I found each other at a breast cancer site shortly after our operations, and her chemo started the day after mine. We e-mailed each other every day through our treatments. We shared our deepest, darkest moments and many tears, but also lots of laughter. In rereading our e-mails, I realise that I shared feelings with Kym that I didn't with my husband, children, or closest friends. I think I put on a good front for those around me, because I wanted to protect them. With Kym, I could express all my concerns. Our e-mails were a safe place for that. Nor were those e-mails all about breast cancer. We talked about our families and shared day-to-day stories. We refused to allow our disease to define or consume us."
Nancy Lane; diagnosed in 2000 at the age of 53; teacher

"I'm the other half of the e-mail penpal duo. Nancy and I literally went through breast cancer treatment together from opposite ends of the country. I initially e-mailed her because I thought I could offer her words of comfort. But Nancy became my comforter, my encouragement. We both had wonderful support systems of family and friends, but we understood everything that was happening to one another in a way that no one else did. I found such comfort in hearing her thoughts, fears and feelings. We shared day-to-day struggles and triumphs. Nancy's strength, wit and compassion gave me courage when I couldn't find any of my own. Even though we have never met, I consider Nancy one of my dearest friends."
Kym Dyer; diagnosed in 2000 at the age of 42; manager

Reciprocity

"While my extended family and friends all knew about my cancer, I didn't share the information with new friends or associates for many years. Then, around 1990, one of the secretaries in my office developed breast cancer and needed a mastectomy. I came out of the closet for her, and it helped both of us. She was strengthened

by seeing my absolutely normal life. And I was strengthened by being able to help someone."
Barbara Jentis; diagnosed in 1983 at the age of 41; lawyer

"Be a mentor to someone newly diagnosed in the same way that you chose a survivor to mentor you. You will be surprised how much value your experience has for others."
Kathy Weaver-Stark; diagnosed in 1991 at the age of 46; loss adjuster, instructor

"Reach out to others. When my sister wasn't in hospital herself, she'd go back to visit other breast cancer patients. Focusing on others made her feel better. Giving regenerated her."
Barbara Keiler; daughter of a survivor

"One of the most rewarding things to come out of my experience with breast cancer is being able to help others. I've had colleagues come to me about people in their lives who have been diagnosed. I'm always glad to be able to help. This is something no one should have to go through alone."
Val Long; diagnosed in 1999 at the age of 47; administrative assistant

"As a professional counsellor I felt that my contribution to the cause could be my willingness to listen and support others. So now I tell friends, family and colleagues that I will talk to anyone they know who is newly diagnosed . . . not to give medical help, but a compassionate ear. Only this past week, I have had two such calls."
Patricia Carr; diagnosed in 1989 at the age of 51; community college professor, counsellor

"I now call on newly diagnosed women and try to be a resource for them. No question is a stupid question. The unknown is one of our worst enemies."
Judy Peterson; diagnosed in 2000 at the age of 58; nurse

"Over the past 11 years, I have had calls from people who know my history, asking me to speak to a friend or loved one of theirs. I always say yes and tell my story. I have been blessed to know that I have helped people get up and move on."
Susan Clemente; diagnosed in 1990 at the age of 46; retired nurse

"Participate in walks or events that promote breast cancer awareness. Give encouragement to others who are undergoing surgery or treatment. Sending a card or making a call may be as therapeutic for you as it will be helpful for them."
Faye Hardiman; diagnosed in 1998 at the age of 50; wife, mother, teacher

"I understood that only someone who had been diagnosed with breast cancer could truly know what I was feeling. I became active in the breast cancer movement. I felt that by going public about what was happening to me and by helping anyone who asked, I was fighting the disease. I started a foundation dedicated to funding research projects which would look at the links between breast cancer and the environment."
Eleanor Anbinder; diagnosed in 1991 at the age of 50; sales manager

"I have embraced my survivor status and have started teaching girls as young as 12 how to examine their breasts. I have helped other cancer patients get through the agony of fighting for their lives. And I have become an avid supporter of breast cancer awareness. I am a breast cancer survivor and I am only 27 years old."
Kimberlee Richardson; diagnosed in 2000 at the age of 26; mother, air force wife, student

"After my diagnosis nine years ago, I decided to do something positive for other women experiencing that scary time in their life. So I became a volunteer in a national cancer society's recovery programme. Doing so has enabled me to meet many wonderful and courageous women."
Susan Sanford; diagnosed in 1992 at the age of 48; retired mortgage insurance underwriter, volunteer

"My mother and her mother both had breast cancer, so I was on the lookout for trouble. I found it in 1981 in the form of a tumour in my left breast. A reoccurrence followed two years later, so by the age of 34, I had had bilateral mastectomies. After the operation, I was visited by a volunteer. She came walking into my house looking fit and healthy, and she was full of energy and so positive it gave me hope. She was what I wanted to be – alive and healthy and strong. So I waited the mandatory year after diagnosis and trained as a

volunteer myself. It has changed my life, just as I know I have changed the lives of the women I visit each month. I am now that picture of health, that strong woman who has beaten breast cancer not once but twice. I now train volunteers. These are women helping women, sharing their experiences as only women can."
Maribeth Stone; diagnosed in 1982 at the age of 32; decorative painting teacher

"About a year ago, I attended my first breast cancer support group meeting. Paul said I was crying in my sleep that night. It costs me to go back to my experience with breast cancer. But I will always try to be there for any woman I meet who is going through any aspect of breast cancer. I have learned, though, that I cannot routinely 'put myself out there' for meetings and still stay calm enough to live my life and do my work."
Jeanne Sturdevant; diagnosed in 1990 at the age of 45; artist

"I decided not to join a breast cancer awareness group, mainly because I have seen it become a hobby with a few women. They walk and talk breast cancer. I had it, it's gone, I want to get on with life. However, I am more willing to discuss it and answer questions for someone who might be going through making all the important decisions."
Lorraine J. Pakkala-Lintala; diagnosed in 1992 at the age of 62; editor, author

"Less than a year after my diagnosis, my daughter was attacked and almost died. My focus immediately switched from me to her. When she went back at college, I was so grateful for both of our lives that I began doing volunteer work at the hospital where I was treated. I needed to give something back. A few years later, I took a part-time job at a cancer information service. Now I can let other women know that they have options and that they shouldn't let fear take over. I am truly blessed."
Marianne Rennie; diagnosed in 1988 at the age of 39; cancer information specialist

"When I heard the words 'You have breast cancer', I knew my life had changed for ever. What I didn't expect was the door that opened for me to make a difference. Three days after my diagnosis,

I met a new friend at a breast cancer support group. We discovered that we lived a street away from each other and exchanged phone numbers. Over the next few months, we talked and checked up on each other, and a special friendship began. Working with our families and a committee of friends, we organised an annual 5km walk/race and a dinner auction. Since then we have raised thousands of pounds for breast cancer research. We now feel that we can do and beat anything."

Cheryl Cavallo; diagnosed in 1997 at the age of 35; housewife

"After surviving two bouts of breast cancer, I realised I needed to give back some of the support and caring that was offered to me. Fortunately, I live in the town where my treatment was taking place. Others were not so lucky. I know that in medical emergencies or during long treatment plans, the last thing you want to think about is where you are going to stay while treatment is going on. Therefore, I thought, why not build a house so much like home that everyone who came to stay could relax and concentrate on regaining their health? After much planning, preparation and building, my dream to 'give back' came true! My 'hospital hospitality house' is seven years old this year and is still going strong!"

Adelaide D. Key; diagnosed in 1978 at the age of 42; community volunteer, philanthropist

11 • Humour

You Have to Laugh . . .

No way, you're thinking, and it's understandable. The last thing you can imagine when you first learn you have breast cancer and become embroiled in the haze of doctor's appointments, treatment schedules and family needs is laughter. After a bit, though, the haze clears. You start adjusting to the reality of the diagnosis – finish making decisions, adapt to a new routine – and your mind isn't as cluttered. Nor is your mouth so busy talking to the world and his wife after that first frenzy. So, that mouth can either turn down, stay flat or turn up. It's your choice.

Survivors opt for the latter. Val Long, who was diagnosed in 1999 at the age of 47, is currently an administrative assistant for a breast cancer charity. She wrote, "Laughter is a big help. Believe it or not, there are a lot of funny things that happen when you're being treated for cancer. Learn to see the funny side. Everything has one."

Asha Mevlana gives a good example of this. A musician, she was diagnosed in 1999 at the age of 24. "Keeping a sense of humour definitely helped me get through the worst. Around the time when my hair started coming out in clumps, my friends and I happened to be out at a restaurant. The food was taking a while, so when the waitress came over, I pretended to get angry. I grabbed my hair with both hands, said I was getting very frustrated that it was taking so long, and pulled huge chunks of hair out in a fit of fake anger. Her mouth dropped. We got our food shortly thereafter."

It isn't just survivors who talk about the importance of humour. Researchers are starting to talk about it, too. While psychologists have long praised humour as a way of decreasing anxiety and stress, more formal studies are showing the actual physiological effects of laughter. Some studies make a connection between laughter and improved circulation and respiration; others suggest that laughter can increase the production of pain-reducing endorphins, or even enhance the immune system. Yet other studies chart a rise in heart rate, circulation and blood pressure during robust laughter, akin to the most beneficial effects of aerobic exercise.

Susan Ragland was diagnosed with breast cancer in 1978, well before these studies were done. She has her own thoughts about laughter, as told in a poignant story.

"In November of 1978, at the age of 45, I was called to the bar. About two weeks later, I found a lump in my breast. I had a mastectomy, followed by 30 days of radiotherapy, which I tolerated well. By now it was early January. There was snow on the ground and I was feeling a cumulative fatigue from the treatments. I asked my husband if we could get away to a warm climate, even for a week, just the two of us. He made the arrangements while I called my neighbour, a travel agent. I said, 'Bess, just get me somewhere where there's sun, where it's warm and where I can just sit and relax. I don't care where it is.' She said that it was a busy time of year, but promised to get to work on it straight away. In the meantime, my sister, also a veteran of breast cancer, took me to buy a mastectomy bathing costume. In those days, the makers of such things must have thought a mastectomy meant that somehow your thighs were injured, because the only decent one they had was high on the chest and skirted to the knee. I was very proud of my legs in those days and wanted to flaunt this remaining sexual asset. But I was going away to a warm climate to recuperate and relax, and I had a loving, caring, attentive husband, who had literally moved heaven and earth to get away on short notice. So I took the swimsuit.

"My travel agent called me back and said, 'You're in luck. I found a small hotel on the French island of Guadaloupe, where there is guaranteed steady sunshine. I think it's just the ticket.' A few days later, encouraged and optimistic, we arrived in the tropics. What a relief, I thought, to escape the dreary, cold, dismal winter.

The only thing I was worried about was my grandma swimming costume. But I said, 'What the hell, who am I here to impress?'

"We went directly to our room. It was lunchtime, and we decided to lunch by the pool and then start relaxing. Reluctantly, I put on my one-piece swimsuit, which was green with white piping (I will never forget that swimsuit, although my husband thought I looked very handsome in it), and went off to the pool to have lunch.

"It was then that it hit me between the eyes. Breasts! Everywhere I looked. Breasts, uncovered, everywhere! There were small ones, large ones, perky young ones, and even some droopy old ones. My travel agent had sent us to a topless hotel and beach! Not only was I the only one covered up, but I had this damn skirt down to my knees. All the good feelings about myself that I'd worked so hard to preserve suddenly vanished.

"My husband started to laugh, and so did I . . . at first. When we got back to the room, I started to cry a flood. My poor husband didn't know what to do. It was funny, it was a scream, but the thought of five more days of this was untenable. No way could I stay there! We got dressed and went to see the hotel manager. He was most sympathetic but informed us that there were only two flights a week in and out of Guadaloupe, and that the next plane out was three days hence. I was trapped. I mustered up my courage and made the best of it, but on the third day we were up early and on that plane. Much to everyone's surprise, we came home, repacked for a cold climate, and went north to our summer home in the mountains, where we made a fire and sat and relaxed and healed. We only had three days there, but I did come home rested – and laughing.

"I am still cancer-free 22-plus years later," she concludes.

Me, I like that punch line the best. But there are other punch lines where humour is concerned. For a sample, read on.

Hair-Ha

"Before cancer, I had bad hair days. After cancer, I had bad hair days, but I could take it off and shake it."
Rosamary Amiet; diagnosed in 2000 at the age of 48; programme manager

"I was standing at the back of our house. I had washed my wig and was shaking out the excess water, thinking that I was alone. I wasn't. Our neighbour's three-year-old daughter yelled, 'Jill, what are you doing?' I said, 'Well, I'm drying my hair.' She looked at me and said, 'My mummy keeps her hair on and uses a machine to dry it.' "

Jill Gross; diagnosed in 2000 at 51; head bank clerk

"When I came home from teaching, I would often take off my wig and put it on a kitchen worktop. If I was distracted, I would go off and leave it there. When Micah (my son) and his friends would come in, I would hear: 'Jane Barnett Royal-Davidson! Get down here this minute!' Being a good mother, I would go downstairs obediently, and there Micah would reprimand me. 'Did my grand-mother Royal teach you to leave your hair on the kitchen worktop? I think not! Did you teach your children to leave their hair on the kitchen worktop? I think not. We take our hair everywhere we go. Now, young lady, I want you to take your hair upstairs to your room and think about what you have done, for, say, at least an hour. Then you may come downstairs and we shall talk.' I would take my hair and go upstairs and lie down for a much-needed nap. Some-times a mother has to do as she is told!"

Jane Royal-Davidson; diagnosed in 1996 at the age of 47; teacher

"I was at a benefit fashion show in my new wig (long, straight auburn hair) when a slightly tipsy gentleman approached me to tell me what lovely hair I had. I smiled politely, thanked him, and went about my business. Every few minutes, he would come back over to me to comment on my hair. Each time he was a little more inebriated and his comments a little more bold. Finally, barely able to stand upright, he slurred, 'I would just love to spend the night running my hands through your lovely red hair.' At this comment, I whipped off my wig, held it out to him, and replied, 'Go on then, I'm going to get a beer.' After picking his jaw up off the ground, he turned on his heel and I never saw him again! I'm sure the next morning, he wondered if that had actually happened or if it was all an alcohol-induced mirage."

Joy West; diagnosed in 2000 at the age of 34; adverstising account co-ordinator

"The day after my operation I got up, drainage tubes and all, went to the sink and washed my hair. The nurse came and, horrified,

said, 'Mrs Abelmann, what are you doing?' My response was, 'I am washing my hair. I do this every morning!' "
Jeryl Abelmann; diagnosed in 1986 at the age of 46; primary school teacher

"One of my best retorts for someone who complimented me on my hair was, 'Thanks – want to borrow it?' "
Rosamary Amiet; diagnosed in 2000 at the age of 48; programme manager

Bra-Ha

"Shortly after my operation, my daughter came to check on me. She felt that I couldn't possibly be doing as well as it seemed from our long-distance phone conversations. We were in the kitchen and she had turned, hitting me on my remaining breast. She said, 'Sorry! At least it was the good one!' My reply? 'It's the *only* one.' I truly believe that keeping a sense of humour is the single most important piece of advice I can share."
Susan Sanford; diagnosed in 1992 at the age of 48; retired mortgage insurance underwriter, volunteer

"After my mastectomy, I rescued a German wire-haired pointer. He was in such need of love, and I was in need of being loved, so we were two lost souls together. One morning I showered at 5.30 a.m. and started to get dressed, only to find that my prosthesis was missing from the side where I'd left it moments before. It took me a few minutes to realise that my dog had it. It smelled like me, so off he'd run with it. I was all over the house chasing this big dog with my prosthesis in his mouth. No matter what I did, he wouldn't let go. I was about to give up and leave him to it, when he dropped it and let me get dressed!"
Jane Royal-Davidson; diagnosed in 1996 at the age of 47; teacher

"Unfortunately, a prosthesis has no sensation. The husband of a friend of mine inadvertently fondled the wrong woman at a cocktail party, and she didn't even know it!"
Mindy Greenside; diagnosed in 2000 at the age of 48; midwife

"Humour is most important. I even had to laugh when a large wave

crashed against me and took my prosthesis out to the coral reefs of Bermuda. I was never self-conscious about my body. I felt that people cared for me for who I am, not what I look like."
Carol Quinn; diagnosed in 1984 at the age of 46; nurse

"I met my Weight Watcher's goal by going into the changing room and removing my breast form. I instantly lost 1¼ pounds."
Helaine Hemingway; diagnosed in 1988 at the age of 41; teacher

"Make 'em laugh! That's what I try to do for friends diagnosed with breast cancer. I sent funny cards, even the Hallmark grumpy old lady with the hanging boobs, to two of my friends who'd just had mastectomies. They both said they laughed heartily, and that it felt great!"
Elaine Raco Chase; friend of many survivors

"Before my implant surgery, I wanted to give my plastic surgeon a unique gift. I needed to outdo his humour for once. The wife of one of my husband's colleagues made me big chocolate breasts, and they were perfect! He loved it! I teased him about using the chocolate breasts for my implant, chocoholic that I was. We took a picture of us holding the breasts. He promised to use the picture on those stressful days when he needed a laugh."
Joanne Palmer; diagnosed in 1996 at the age of 42; medical receptionist

Happy Face

"Bubble baths were soothing and relaxing. But the best medicine was to laugh as often as possible."
Carol Snyder; diagnosed in 1992 at the age of 47; special needs teacher

"The best advice I got was from Nanny, my friend Julie's grandmother, who was a 45-year survivor of a double mastectomy: 'Just keep on doing the laundry!' "
Betsy Goree; diagnosed in 1998 at the age of 40; magazine publisher/editor

"A sense of humour will make the dark days manageable and fun."
Susan Clemente; diagnosed in 1990 at the age of 46; retired nurse

"The best thing about cancer? I am healthier, funnier and nicer

than I was before. Now I run, I gave up drinking wine and I've just taken a year off work to live in style. I really get it now. Life is short – eat dessert first!"
Sharon Carr; diagnosed in 1997 at the age of 42; hospice grief counsellor

"It's a lot better to laugh than to feel sorry for yourself. Go fishing, play cards, do anything to take your mind off yourself."
Billie Loop; diagnosed in 1997 at the age of 63; housewife

"I got out of hospital on a Thursday. On Friday, two friends came and bathed my Newfoundlands, and we were all at the dog show on Sunday. People kept running up to my friend asking how I was and whether I was out of hospital. 'Out of hospital, hell, she's sitting over there!' "
Lynne Rutenberg; diagnosed in 1980 at the age of 35; retired teacher

"My private joke about tattooing the breast for radiation? I'm single and looking for a boyfriend to play join the dots!"
Cindy Ferus; diagnosed in 2000 at the age of 57; circuit board technician, former schoolteacher

"On the lighter side, when you have cancer, you try to laugh. Three weeks before my mastectomy, my mother and I meet a plastic surgeon. I pretend I am in Hollywood. I am Cher, who's come in for a facelift. The doctor swivels his chair towards my mother. 'So you're considering reconstruction?' I cut in. 'Wait. It's not her. It's me.' Swivelling in my direction without missing a beat, he starts again. 'So you're considering reconstruction?' "
Carol Dine; diagnosed in 1980 at the age of 36; college professor, writer

"Humour was most important in helping me survive this ordeal. While my husband was shaving my head and calling me Kojak, I was telling him what a bargain I was, since the family budget for haircare products had just been cut in half!"
Renee C. Johannesen; diagnosed in 1993 at the age of 35; marketing communications manager

Smile and the World Smiles . . .

"I was pregnant with my second child when diagnosed. I had a

mastectomy while I was eight months pregnant and started chemotherapy when my son was one week old. Friends brought us dinner every night – a lifesaver – and the dozens of cards, notes and phone calls I received were very uplifting, as was keeping my sense of humour. A close friend, upon hearing of my diagnosis, said in all seriousness, 'Feel free to call if there's anything you need to get off your chest.' I said, 'Actually, I'd rather not!' which gave us a good laugh."
Laurie Bishop; diagnosed in 1998 at the age of 40; housewife, mother

"When I told my friend Liesel that I had been diagnosed with breast cancer and was going to have a double mastectomy, she asked me if I was planning to have prostheses made. No one else had asked this, so I asked why. With a twinkle in her eye, Liesel sat me down on one of her elegant fur throws and told me about a friend of hers. Apparently, there is a dressmaker in Chicago who had prostheses made out of her pincushions, so that she could conveniently stick her needles and pins into her chest when sewing and making alterations!"
Darlene Jurow; diagnosed in 1995 at the age of 52; interior designer

"My son, Wil, was five when I was diagnosed. I explained my mastectomy and reconstructive surgery to him by saying that I had a 'boo-boo' in my chest that my doctor would cut out and that he would put great big Band-Aids on the cuts. Wil was not bothered by my actual surgery but by the fact that my Band-Aids didn't have Pokémon on them.

"For a long while after the operation, I could only wear sports bras. One day, while I was dressing, Wil came running up carrying my sports bra. He announced, 'Mummy! Here is your booby trap!'

"Before chemo, I explained to Wil that I was going to have to take some medicine that would make my hair fall out. I explained that I would wear a wig, which I described as a hat with hair. A week later, we were in a bookshop ordering children's books on cancer. One of the titles was something like 'My Mummy Has No Hair'. Wil piped up, 'That's okay. My mummy is going to wear a hairy hat!' "
Joy West; diagnosed in 2000 at the age of 34; advertising account co-ordinator

"I have a rowing friend who is also a gifted jeweller. At my 50th birthday party, I opened her present, and it was a gold stud ear-ring mounted with a diamond. The card was sweet and sentimental. It ended with 'P.S. I am so sorry for your loss, but they make them in gold now.' I thanked her graciously. At 4 a.m. the next day, I sat up in bed and realised that the stud was a gold breast with a diamond nipple! Apparently the other guests at the party had thought I was embarrassed and had let the joke drop. I wear this ear-ring with pride and never think of taking it off."

Diane Cotting; diagnosed in 1999 at the age of 49; insurance broker

"People said some strange things to me during the time I was undergoing treatment and shortly afterwards. For example, when my hair first returned, it was jet black instead of the lighter brown it had been before chemo. One asked, 'Is that your hair? I don't believe it. Are you sure that's your hair?' "

Fran DiBiase; diagnosed in 1994 at the age of 40; part-time teacher, part-time property management

"My best friend and her family decided to go on holiday during one of her three-week rotations of chemotherapy. She had the first round at home and took the second with her to her destination. When she walked into the hospital where the chemo was to be given, she was met by a young intern. As he was hooking her up he asked, 'Why in heaven's name did you decide to remove your breast?' Janey replied, 'I am a world-class archer, and it just got in the way.' He asked no more questions."

Judy Bayha; Janey's friend

"It's funny. It's almost as though another woman was living inside me and revealed herself just when I needed her. All my life, I had been a prude about undressing in front of other people. But I understood that undressing would be part of the process and my modesty just seemed to disappear. In fact, I told one of the nurses that I needed to be careful at work, because every time I walked into a small office, I felt the urge to take off my clothes."

Val Long; diagnosed in 1999 at the age of 47; administrative assistant

"To get through radiotherapy, I reached for humour. When I rang my mother to tell her the number of treatments had been reduced, I explained that it just takes less time to cook a small pot roast. Friends helped me create humour. For example, there were monitors outside the radiotherapy room. When I mentioned this to my brother, he said that was why there were satellite dishes on the top of the hospital – so the image of me lying there with one breast hanging out could be broadcast everywhere. When I relayed this story to a friend, he carried it further, launching into a conversation between two Martians in a spaceship pointing to the image of me on their radar screen. Whenever I thought of this image, I would laugh – even in the middle of a treatment."

Jeanne Sturdevant; diagnosed in 1990 at the age of 45; artist

"My son had planned to marry several weeks before Christmas. Then I was diagnosed with breast cancer. He offered to postpone the wedding, but I told him to proceed. A week before the event, I had my lymph node dissection. On the day of the wedding, I was horrified to find that the drainage tube had fallen out. There was no time for the doctor to put another one in. All I could see was me walking down the aisle of the church with lymph drainage all over my beautiful new dress. So I came up with an idea. I placed a sanitary pad over my surgical site, then put on my bra so it would hold the pad in place. Then I had my husband wrap my body in clingfilm. I walked down the aisle, with no drainage in sight, and thoroughly enjoyed the reception. That night when I undressed and unwound the clingfilm, I found there was no drainage at all. The surgical site was stopped up. I laughed, thinking that I now knew what a chicken felt like after being wrapped in clingfilm."

Voncile Jones; diagnosed in 1994 at the age of 54; nurse

"A telesalesman rang me called me one afternoon: 'Good afternoon, Jane, and how are you?' So I told him. I said that I had recently been diagnosed with breast cancer. I had had a lumpectomy, which had been scheduled to enable me to keep my promise to help my juniors revise before their exam – and, of course, it had to fit in with my summer teaching schedule, and there was Micah's first professional gig with his band. Then my surgeon had decided they needed a cleaner margin, so I had to have a mastectomy, which had to fit around my teaching, too. And there was the decision about what type of chemotherapy to have, and Micah to get off to Israel and Louis to summer school and Douglas to camp. There were also the flowers that I needed to get into the garden and then I really needed to get a haircut before all of my hair fell out. 'So that is how I am,' I told the man. 'How can I help you?' He stuttered, and then asked if all of that was true. I asked to be removed from his list, wished him a nice day and hung up. Louis and Douglas were listening to all this, literally rolling on the floor. Telesalespeople didn't ring us for ages."

Jane Royal-Davidson; diagnosed in 1996 at the age of 47; teacher

"When people around you hear the 'C' word, it rocks their world. Once they recover from the shock, odds are they will ask, 'How are you?' followed by the inevitable 'Let me know if there's anything I can do.' After hearing that again and again, I decided to take those who offered at their word. I told them what I needed. And what I needed was to laugh. Instead of crying, or whining, or feeling sorry for myself and asking 'Why me?' I needed to laugh. After all, I'd had a sense of humour before I was diagnosed. I wanted it back. So I asked those near and dear to me to send me things to make me laugh. And, lo and behold, they did. My 'laughter therapy' arrived in different shapes and forms. It included a book of rants, a videotape of a family member at a comedy club open mike night, photocopies of funny cartoons, a T-shirt with the words 'Bite me' on it, Woody Allen short stories, shipments of cat beanie babies and rainbow-coloured socks with individual toes. Now, cards are sweet and flowers smell good. But in my book, when you are feeling alone and down and somewhat tragic dealing with a health crisis, nothing's better than opening a surprise parcel from a dear friend or family member. And if you rip open the package and it makes you smile from ear to ear, well, that is what I call healing medicine for the soul."

Alysa Cummings; diagnosed in 1998 at the age of 45; educational trainer

12 • Men

By, For and About

Men play a role in our lives. They may be family members, as in fathers, husbands or sons. They may be significant others. They may be simply friends. Or bosses. Any one of these roles puts them prominently into the breast cancer picture. Survivors mention them often – so often, in fact, that I wanted to know more.

Now that might surprise you. After all, I have a husband and three sons, and we're a close family. So I should know how men feel and what they need during this time, right?

Wrong. Because when you're living it, you don't want to talk about fears. You have your hands full dealing with a busy daily life made even busier by breast cancer. Touchy-feely stuff, sensitive stuff, stuff that shows vulnerabilities and foibles, that's sometimes just too slippery to grasp. You satisfy yourself by knowing that actions speak louder than words.

You finish treatment, regain strength and life quietens down. Time passes. You move beyond breast cancer. Then something happens – say, *UPLIFT* – and it suddenly occurs to you to wonder what they were thinking and feeling back then. So you ask. You ask them separately, so they won't feel as though they have to compete with each other for answers. And each of the four, on his own, does pretty much the same thing. He shrugs. He gives a mystified little smile. 'It wasn't any big deal,' he says. 'You were confident. You promised you'd tell us everything. You never really missed a beat.'

Oh, there were other little memories. Tears on the phone. A hug when that was the only thing that brought comfort. Festive holidays. Special Valentines. Lopsided breasts at a graduation.

My husband swears that he was never frightened. 'Never?' I ask him, wondering if I should be disappointed, worried, offended. He shakes his head, as quiet and sure as he's ever been, and it strikes me that we all shared the very same view of my breast cancer. From the start, death was simply not an option.

Those were my men, dealing with our situation in keeping with our own family dynamics. But just as the survivors were proving to be a widely diverse group, I knew that their men would be, too. I wanted to hear from those men – wanted to know how they felt when a woman in their life was diagnosed, how they learned about the disease, to whom they talked, who gave them comfort. I wanted to know what advice they would give other men in the same situation – other men who might, just might, pick up UPLIFT when they needed a boost.

So I sent an e-mail to each of the women who had already become part of UPLIFT and asked if they would try to convince the men in their lives to submit a thought or two. Talk about opening floodgates. Based on the immediacy of their replies, these men were thrilled to have a chance to speak!

Take Marvin Wilker, who says, "When Helen told me she had breast cancer, I felt as though I'd been hit by a ten-ton truck." And Bryan Whittet, who writes, "When my wife was first diagnosed, I was devastated." And George Anbinder, whose first thoughts "were ones of disbelief and denial". And that's only the start. These three and many others have much more to say about breast cancer, not the least inspiring being Dave Schwingel, who wrote about his wife, Gracie, "Cancer has changed her. She is more independent, self-assured and free. But never alone."

This one's for you, guys. It may validate things you've been feeling. It may give you ideas about where to turn and what to do. It'll certainly tell you that you're not alone.

He Says: What I felt

"The day of my wife's operation, I went to hospital with her. When

the doctor came out halfway through to tell me that the lump had tested malignant and he would remove her breast, I was instantly scared to death. My brother went out to the car with me, where I spent the last part of her surgery crying. I was so afraid she would die. A couple of years later, when she had a biopsy on the other breast, one of our sons sat with me while I cried again. That was almost ten years ago. I have never entirely lost my fear of her dying, but my strength and comfort have always come from my wife. She trusted her doctors and her treatment. We made it through together."
Robert David Vaughan, Jane's husband

"When my wife was first diagnosed, I was devastated. We both cried, but I knew I had to calm her down. Our families gave us comfort . . . and, of course, our kids. My advice to other men? Support whatever your wife decides to do, and be patient. Having the breast removed may be the easy part; the emotional aftermath may be more of a struggle."
Bryan Whittet, Debby's husband

"I was only 17 years old, away from home for the first time and in my first term at college when my mum told me she had breast cancer. I couldn't stop the tears. I thought she was going to die. After my parents left to go home, I went out with some friends and got drunk for the first time! Then I talked to my friends. Three guys I lived with all had a story about someone in their lives who'd had breast cancer and beat it, so that helped me a lot. My parents rang every day to see how I was. When I told my mum that I was going to come home to help her, she said, 'No. Stay at college and do the best you can. That will be all the help I need.' I got straight As that term! I would advise other kids to treat their mums just like they did before. I always made her laugh, and I went back to college thinking she was going to be okay, and she was."
Brandon Whittet, Debby's son

"When Helen told me she had breast cancer, I felt as though a ten-ton truck had run over me. I remember feeling helpless, feeling that there was nothing I could do to change anything but pray, and pray I did. I wanted to cry but held back the tears. I didn't want her worrying about me; she had enough on her mind. At work, I sometimes broke down, and my colleagues comforted me. The person who helped me the most was the surgeon when he said that Helen's chance of full recovery was excellent. I would advise other men in my position to hang in there, think positive thoughts and look for that light at the end of the tunnel. Who said 'Life is fair'? Not I."

Marvin Wilker, Helen's husband

" 'Knowing about' becomes 'knowing of'. Learning more about cancer, healing, food, exercise, the spirit and alternatives were all pivotal to Grace's decisions. I am there when she needs personal support – an ear to listen, an eye to see, lips to smile, a shoulder to lean on, arms to hug her and a heart to support her always."

Dave Schwingel, Gracie's husband

"As the husband of a cancer patient my part has been very limited. I only had to be there on the bad days, and with Kathleen's attitude, those were few and far between. My advice to other men? Don't ever treat the disease with any other thought but total recovery."

Richard Griffith, Kathleen's husband

"My first thoughts were ones of disbelief and denial, but these rapidly changed when we met the doctors. Ellie's first surgical appointment was with a cold, unfeeling male surgeon. I immediately secured an appointment with a well-known and respected female surgeon. She provided much comfort. I remember most clearly how well Ellie dealt with the entire situation."

George Anbinder, Eleanor's husband

"When I first heard my wife's diagnosis, I was frightened for her. Having had combat surgery, I had a sense of what she faced. Christine's doctors gave me all the confidence that I could ever have hoped for. I remember the calm, cool way the surgeon told us how he would approach the surgery, and how he respected Christine's judgement. That first office visit set the tone for everything that followed. All men whose loved ones have breast cancer should meet the doctors so that they are in on the direction of the treatment, almost as they would be at the birth of a child."

Denis McNamara, Christine's husband

"When I first heard that my partner, Dorian, had breast cancer, I felt absolute, complete, utter shock. I'm the type of person who worries and works hard to make sure nothing goes wrong. I double-check that my front door is locked before I go to bed. I always wear a seatbelt. I eat healthy food. To have my partner diagnosed with breast cancer at the age of 26 was something I couldn't even imagine, a risk I had never prepared for. It still feels almost surreal. The time we spent in a support group for young adults with cancer and their partners was a really transformative experience. The counsellor made it clear that if we husbands and partners attended the group with an I'm-just-here-to-support-my-partner attitude, we'd be missing out. Breast cancer affects the whole family, especially partners. It threw into question some of my unspoken and even unquestioned beliefs about health and sickness, life and mortality. Being in a group with other people in their twenties and thirties meant a lot to us. As men we're brought up to think that it's our job to solve problems. And many of us *are* really good problem-solvers. But sometimes with breast cancer there's just nothing we can do. That can be the hardest thing of all: knowing that the woman you so love and care about has breast cancer – and you're utterly powerless to do anything about it. It's not your job to come up with the magical solution and tell her how to fix it. All you can do is support her and be by her side."
Marshall Miller, Dorian Solot's partner

"My first thoughts on learning that my 26-year-old daughter had breast cancer? Disbelief, shock, anger and denial. There was grief, then acceptance, then the commitment to research and pursue all avenues. Since most research and treatment has been on older women, we felt it was important to consider the long-term effects on a young woman with many years of life ahead of her. I talked about it to everyone, passing what they had to offer on to Dorian. The support was overwhelming. I felt guilty about the outpouring of love for me, which I believed should have been directed exclusively to Dorian. I've come to understand and appreciate that support and how it continues to buoy us up. It was wonderful to receive so many calls that it was necessary to allocate whose return call would have to be put off. Ultimately, the greatest comfort came from Dorian herself. I knew that her diligent research, combined with her intelligence and intuition, would lead her to the correct decisions, whether or not they aligned with prevailing practice. Also, knowing that Marshall (her wise and wonderful partner) would be there for her was a tremendous relief. Single moments: seeing her in hospital after the first procedure, and feeling the wonder of the fragility/strength balance. Also, having the twisted privilege of being able to take care of her for a few days as she recovered – a treat for me, connecting her childhood to the present – a reminder of our father/daughter/friend relationship and how it continues to evolve. Advice to other men: place her unique individuality first. Sift through the books and advice with *her* in mind, looking and listening for her needs. Holding hands is good for both of you."

Evan Solot; Dorian's father

"When my 26-year-old granddaughter told us of her diagnosis, I was convinced there was an error. I couldn't associate breast cancer with the child we nurtured and loved. How could we spare her the agony or any pain? How could I sit quietly by to let her make her decisions for her survival? It was difficult for me to discuss this with my male friends, but I was able to discuss this with female friends, who have offered much support. Gradually, Dorian convinced me that hope is there for us, that her remission continues and that her recovery will be full and complete with the regimen she is following. Her positive approach to her recovery has helped me through this unbelievable event."

Leslie Solot, Dorian's grandfather

"A woman facing mastectomy, particularly a young woman, might want to videotape herself before surgery. I know this may sound a little ghoulish, but it might be helpful. It is something to share with a current or future lover. I speak as a guy. Sometimes we can't imagine what we can't see. It's often easier to empathise when one knows what has been lost. I don't minimise the value our society places on women's breasts. Even so, there are men who are not breast obsessed. Breast cancer survivors need to know that. A woman's life is so much more than the quantity and positioning of a little bit, or even a lot, of flesh. Breasts don't laugh, smile, share brilliance or give kindness. Life is the true treasure; otherwise, we'd save the breast and discard the woman. A living woman is beautiful. A dead woman is not nearly so attractive. For the record, I am 42, and I really like women."

Alan S. Gardner; no relation to anyone with breast cancer, just an all-round good person

"I fell in love with my wife one year after her diagnosis. Part of what attracted me to Cathleen was her strength and her determination to beat the disease after being diagnosed before she was 30 years old. She was so vibrant and full of life that I immediately fell in love with her. About two months after we were married, they discovered a recurrence. This was devastating. Here we had just married, ready to begin our lives together, and the disease reared its ugly head. However, together we attacked this as just a bump in the road. We are forever optimists, insisting that it is better we caught this early. I look at my wife and all she has gone through, and I tell myself that she is one of a kind."
Mark D'Antonio, Cathleen's husband

"My wife Billie prayed about herself and her breast cancer, and when the doctor had to remove her breast, she couldn't understand why for a while. But we talked about it. I told her I didn't care about her breast. I cared about her. It has been four years now, and everything is going fine. She is still beautiful in my sight. We just celebrated our 50th anniversary. We are friends, lovers and best pals. There is no one in the world I would rather be with. I call her Sug."
Donald Loop, Billie's husband

She Says: What He Felt

"My husband's first reaction to my diagnosis was shock. He talks about it with friends and people at work, and all have been extremely supportive. They ask how I'm doing, but also how he's doing, and that makes me feel good. I think it is important to take care of our mates as much as ourselves. His advice to other men? Be there for her. Let her talk, cry, whine, shout – whatever makes her feel better. Go to all her appointments with her, even if it means sitting around being bored. Reassure her that a mastectomy is not the end of the world. Tell her 'I love you – two breasts, one breast, or no breasts.' Most of all, repeatedly tell her that we will get through this, and that she is going to live a long, long time."
Lori Bartz; diagnosed in 2000 at the age of 41; customer service representative

"Whenever my friend Eunice Silverstein went to the gynaecologist for her yearly tests, her husband, Stan, worried. Eunice is the youngest of five sisters, three of whom had already had breast cancer. Though all three were survivors, when Eunice was finally diagnosed herself, Stan was very frightened. But he decided he had to put a good face on it, with positive thoughts and comments to Eunice. He felt that fear was contagious, and he didn't want Eunice to catch his fear when she had enough of her own to contend with. So he stayed calm, and discussed his worries only with Eunice's sisters, since they had been through this together. It was a shared family experience. Eunice has been cancer-free now for more than 15 years."

Rae Shapiro; friend of Stan and Eunice Silverstein

My husband's first reaction was shock. He felt lost, not knowing what to say or do. Then he sat down with me and told me that it didn't matter if I had one or two breasts, because that's not what he married me for. He told me we would get through this together. He took me to get my chemo treatments and made dinner when I couldn't – and he's a good cook! When I came home from hospital, he didn't want to see my scar. This scared me a little. Then, the next day he did look at it, because he realised what it meant to me for him to see it. Then there was the day he touched it and found it to be just fine. Cancer is tough stuff, but love is stronger."

Mary Ann Budnick; diagnosed in 1991 at the age of 44; school bus driver

"I asked my son Tom, who lives a long way away, what he felt when I was first diagnosed. He said, 'I can't remember exactly how I found out about it, but I do remember not being too worried. I know that sounds strange, but I knew that you had a good attitude and good doctors. I just knew you would be okay. Obviously, I was concerned about you having surgery, and was prepared to come and help you, but I looked at this as one of life's lessons and nothing that we would not get over. I remember thinking that we should never be too cocky about all the good things God gives us. I remember thinking that this was His way of keeping us a bit humble.' "

Ann Gordon; diagnosed in 1998 at the age of 73; retired business executive

"My oldest male friend, Terry, who has taught with me for 26 years, said that his first reaction was fear – fear on many levels. He couldn't imagine the stress and turmoil that I would be in; he imagined himself and his wife in the same situation and tried to figure out what he could say that would support me and give me encouragement. My friend Dickie was scared for me, too, because his mum had succumbed to cancer years ago, when detection and treatment were not at the level that they are now. Once he calmed down, he was totally optimistic. Mike is my chiropractor and a good friend. He was confident that I was getting the best care and that my mental attitude was very positive."

Christine Foutris; diagnosed in 1999 at the age of 49; teacher

"My husband was as grateful as I was for the support of friends and family. His advice to other men: 'Be patient and understanding during the post-surgery treatment. Chemo and radiotherapy can be physically exhausting and emotionally draining.' "

Brenda M. Kraft; diagnosed in 1986 at the age of 60; retired schoolteacher

Dialogues

"I felt my lump on Palm Sunday. I thought it ironic that as things grew in the spring, cancer was growing in my breast. I remember looking out at the daffodils and saying to my family, 'Next year, as we watch the flowers come up, this will all be behind us.' "

Jacki Anthony; diagnosed in 1998 at the age of 48; nurse

"When I first learned about my wife's breast cancer, I felt anger and fear. I was a police officer in a major city, and I was lost at first. Then I went online to cancer sites and read anything I could get my hands on. The information – some good, some bad – was very helpful to me. I went with my wife to every appointment and spoke to the doctors about the procedure, the treatment, and the possibilities. The end results were very good."

Robert Anthony, Jacki's husband

"My family was very supportive, and in turn I was honest with them about everything that needed to be discussed. My husband and his ice hockey team were my biggest fans. They dedicated the season and the championship tournament to me, and skated over to me with the biggest trophy I had ever seen. How could I possibly ever forget that moment?"

Jacki Anthony

"When my team won the championship, they skated over to my wife and presented her with the game trophy and game puck. This was something we did not expect but will always remember."
Robert Anthony

"I was at a conference and with friends when Nina called me to say that she had breast cancer. The friends were a husband and wife. The wife gave me the most assurance that things would be okay, and the husband was supportive, too. The person who gave me the most strength and comfort through all this, though, was Nina. She is a very strong lady and has a great positive attitude."
Roger James, Nina Miller's husband

"My fiancé and I bought a house together in November 1996. In December I found a lump. When we learned it was malignant, we had to decide about the wedding – whether to cancel it, postpone it, move the date forward, or plan it around hair loss and therapy. We decided to wait until treatment was over, but there was no question of waiting for my hair to grow back. I decided to cut back on work during my radiotherapy. I took my afternoons off to plan the wedding. Two weeks after radiation was over, we had a wonderful, personal ceremony in our church's chapel and a reception with friends and family in the garden of our new home."
Nina Miller; diagnosed in 1997 at the age of 40; manager, oncology social worker

"We gave each other a lot of strength through those early days and through the days of treatment. We also had a strong faith in God that helped us through, and a vicar who was quite comforting. The thing I remember the most was the early helpless feeling and the thoughts that Nina was going to die, but the longer she goes without problems, the less we think about that. The advice I'd give others is that this diagnosis is not a death sentence and that one has to be positive and take control of the situation."
Roger James

"When I lost my hair and decided to have it shaved off to avoid the mess, well, that was hard. But then my husband gave me the most wonderful gift of love. He had his head shaved too, so I would not have to go through this alone."

Dee Pobjoy; diagnosed in 1999 at the age of 41; sales clerk

"It was very traumatic for my wife when she lost her hair. I will never forget her surprise when I had my head shaved too. She was speechless, and let me tell you, Dee is never speechless! When she was first diagnosed with breast cancer, I was in shock. Then, all I wanted to do was to hold her and reassure her that she would not be alone in this. My advice to other men? This is not the end of the world, guys. Show your loved one how much you love her, and the rest is easy."

Al Pobjoy, Dee's husband

"When they told me I had cancer, I just shut down. After the surgery, I remembered what a friend had told me: 'I have breast cancer, but it doesn't have me.' I kept telling myself that. To me, it was all in the attitude. I am fine now. Yes, I live in fear that it will come back, but if it does, well, I have this experience to give me hope. A positive attitude is just the most important part of dealing with breast cancer."

Dee Pobjoy

"Dee has shown remarkable strength through all of this. She had surgery for breast cancer and was back at work less than a week later. She would have a chemo treatment and would only miss a day of work. Yes, she has cried – so have I – but she has continued to show strength in the most difficult situations. I admire my wife so much."

Al Pobjoy

"My biggest challenge when my wife went through breast cancer was knowing how to offer support. My instincts in this regard – to be dispassionate and offer advice – weren't always helpful. What worked was to ask Deb what she wanted me to do, and to keep this in mind when she needed help. I had a full repertoire of responses, but matching them to Deb's situation was a challenge. The payoff was the good feeling of doing the right thing during a crisis for someone I loved."

Curt Lamb, Deborah Pierce's husband

"My doctors gave me the option of different treatments. This forced me to do some research. At times the task seemed insurmountable. I was not an expert in the field and was too involved to see clearly."
Deborah Pierce; diagnosed in 1997 at the age of 48; architect

"One of the things I did which Deb appreciated was to read through some of the very technical reports she received to help her make sense of them."
Curt Lamb

"This helped me to take responsibility for decisions, so that I never felt forced into something that wasn't right for me."
Deborah Pierce

"I work in a veterans' hospital, and while I am in the administrative department, I have learned much about the advances of medicine. Still, it made my stomach drop when we heard the news. A supervisor of mine at the time advised me to give Jeanne all the support I could and to be with her throughout this period, and I was. We had good supportive friends and this helped me as much as it did her. I think the hardest part was seeing the frustration, even occasional misery, that she went through. It was hard not being able to do anything to help her."
Paul E. Sturdevant, Jeanne's husband

"My husband has a deep and continuing interest in my physical well-being. Every time I get good reports, he is relieved and satisfied. He almost seems to spin on his heels as he goes on to resume his activities. Even so many years later, I need him to stand there and listen to me talk through my emotions and fears. It may cost him a lot to engage on that visceral level, but that is the level I'm on."
Jeanne Sturdevant; diagnosed in 1990 at the age of 45; artist

"On the way home from hospital, still shocked by the diagnosis and the choice I had to make between lumpectomy and mastectomy, I said to my husband, 'If I have the breast cut off, perhaps I could make it an offering, a sacrifice of old things in return for a new life?' That evening, on the back of an old desk calendar, he drew

an outline of a lateral view of my breasts. In the centre was a black dot – the cancer – with lines that radiated to the edges of the breast. On the side, he wrote, 'All negative energy be gone in the breast of Christine!' Over the next two weeks, I wrote down on this diagrammatic outline all of the negative emotion, the rage, the fear and despair. I finished the night before surgery. It was amazing to see all that stuff out there, outside me. I was ready to let it go, to let go of the breast that contained the essence of all that pain."
Christine McNamara; diagnosed in 2000 at the age of 54; retired doctor

"I told everyone we knew that Christine had cancer. I didn't want it to be a secret just between us. I wanted to use everyone's positive energy to help us face it. Christine's doctors gave me confidence; I felt they were supermen who could do anything. I remember the calm, cool way the surgeon told us how he would approach the surgery, and how he respected Christine's judgement with regard to her own treatment and destiny. That first office visit set the tone for everything that followed. I think it's important for men in the same position to meet the doctors, so that they are in on the direction of the treatment. I also advise them to be completely honest about the fear that they have. For me there was no real fear, due to my having had combat surgery, but I think open discussion really helps."
Denis McNamara, Christine's husband

"I am a male breast cancer survivor. Nine years ago, I had a modified radical mastectomy and underwent chemotherapy. Because I found the lump early, my prognosis is very good."
David Kingsley; diagnosed in 1991 at the age of 44; lawyer

"When my father was diagnosed with breast cancer, I could not believe it. What he underwent has transformed the way I perceive situations. The meaninglessness of problems comes into perspective when I compare them to what we have overcome. Our family survived a battle that was won by my father's immeasurable courage. We all clutch at the hope that life will be fair, yet when it is not, we are awakened. We seek an explanation from somewhere, anywhere. There is none. But I did not become a pessimist. I did not let the disease win. I let it teach me to appreciate everything I once accepted as a given. Life is a gift."
Linda Kingsley, David's daughter

"I am, to my knowledge, the only male breast cancer volunteer in my area, maybe the whole country. I answer telephone calls from around the country, as well as seeing men in my geographical area. I think it's important for people to know that breast cancer does also strike men and that early detection and treatment are a necessity."
David Kingsley

And for Dessert – Mars Bars

"My husband is my lifeline. Even when I had no hair and was so sick, he held me and told me I was beautiful."
Kathy Rabassa; diagnosed in 1999 at the age of 34; administrative assistant

"My husband's support was priceless. He changed my drainage dressing without even making a face – though I can't change a Band-Aid for him without moaning and groaning. Also, he is a very private person, yet he walked in a breast cancer sponsored walk with me. Then I signed up to be in a trial programme to discuss the emotional effect of breast cancer on your family, without realising that he needed to go with me. He agreed because he knew I wanted to do it. We both got a lot out of it."
Sheila Roper; diagnosed in 1995 at the age of 57; housewife

"Before I was diagnosed, my husband and I were beginning to drift apart. I often consider that my having had breast cancer was a gift, because the experience brought us closer together. It gave us a true appreciation of life, and we began enjoying each other much more. We came to realise what is important and what isn't. My husband was so happy that I survived that he became attuned to my needs. We were able to enjoy a much richer and deeper relationship."
Sheila Steinhauser; diagnosed in 1985 at the age of 41; office manager

"What made me feel the most feminine was the fact that my husband wanted to have sex with me."
Frances Gallello; diagnosed in 2000 at the age of 51; mental health assistant

"Sex during treatment – that's is a good idea. Both of you may cry the first time, but sex will leave you feeling normal. It will make you

realise that life goes on, and it's a jumpstart to getting used to your new body image."
Betsy Goree; diagnosed in 1998 at the age of 40; magazine publisher/editor

"My whole treatment programme lasted a school year – from September to early summer. On the last day of treatment, my husband took me out for lunch and gave me a rose!"
Fran DiBiase; diagnosed in 1994 at the age of 40; part-time teacher, part-time property management

"When my daughter-in-law first told me about *UPLIFT*, I felt that I couldn't contribute. It's been three years since my surgery, and with the exception of the day when I learned that my tumour was indeed malignant, the rest of the time has been only good and positive. What more could I say? Then the letter came asking me about the men in my life, and I knew what to write. The love of my life – my husband of 53 years – is the reason why my experience with breast cancer was a positive one. When I was given the diagnosis, he held me and told me that he loved me, no matter what might happen, and that we would go through this together. Luke and our kids are my personal support group. I thank God every day for their love. My recovery has been so easy!"
Ellen R. Luecke; diagnosed in 1998 at the age of 71; retired

"The contract with my husband, my partner is very important
Be honest about everything, tell him everything
Get him to go to the doctor and treatments
Tell him how it feels to go for tests and treatments
He will understand
He stands by me and I stand by him
Together, he says, we can go through anything."
Ruth Jones; diagnosed in 1985 at the age of 51; housewife

"My husband tried to balance every trip to the doctor's office or treatment with a fun stop either before or after. Either we stopped for a cup of coffee, or we went into a bookshop to browse or we went for an ice cream. I almost began to look forward to chemo days!"
Vivian; diagnosed in 1998 at the age of 36; professor

"My husband was wonderful. He took over the household chores, was with me for every treatment and every up-and-down swing. We'd make Fridays our Fun Day after each treatment. We went out for lunch, treats and day trips. I found myself looking forward to going to my treatment appointments because of our outings."
Alyce Feinstein; diagnosed in 1993 at the age of 58; administrative assistant

"The most touching, sweet thing happened to me during those try-ing days when I looked like one of those hairless aliens who stepped off the mother ship in *Close Encounters*. I'd just stepped out of the shower and looked in the mirror to find that the last stringy hair on my head had finally disappeared, when my husband of 35 years tapped at the door. He'd never seen me bald; I'd worn a wig during the day and a turban to bed, because I was insecure about my looks. Well, I wrapped my head in a towel and let him inside. I don't know why I finally did it, but suddenly I decided to just take the stupid towel off my head, and I immediately started to cry. Mike held me, smiled right into my lashless eyes and said, 'So what?' And I thought the best I'd ever hear from him was 'I love you.' "
Lauren Nichols; diagnosed in 2000 at the age of 53; writer

"I am married to the eternal optimist. When I asked what he thought when I first told him I had breast cancer, he said, 'I knew everything was going to be okay!' My having cancer was a double whammy, since he had been diagnosed with prostate cancer just six months before. We dealt with mine the same way we had with his. He had been such a good patient that I couldn't complain much. By the way, we're both doing fine. My last mammogram was nega-tive, the hot flushes are lessening and his PSAs have all been nega-tive! We have much to be thankful for. And for Christmas, he surprised me with a cruise. We leave next month. We're celebrat-ing 37 years of a wonderful life together!"
Judy Peterson; diagnosed in 2000 at the age of 58; nurse

"At Christmas, after I had finished treatments, my husband gave me a gorgeous ring of rubies and diamonds. He explained that the rubies represented adriamycin (the red devil from chemo) and the diamonds represented cytoxin, which is clear. This ring is a fabu-lous 'reward' for all I went through, and I strongly suggest that

other husbands follow mine's lead. This beautiful ring is less a reminder of my cancer treatment than it is a reminder of how lucky I am to have the love and support of this wonderful man."
Nancy Lane; diagnosed in 2000 at the age of 53; teacher

"The day of my last treatment, my husband's company gave him a surprise retirement party. My daughter and I stood at the back, and as he came in, before acknowledging anyone, he came over and kissed me."
Barbara C. Sumner; diagnosed in 1982 at the age of 59; housewife

"The best thing that ever happened to me happened while I was battling breast cancer: my boyfriend, whom I had been dating for seven years, proposed to me when I looked my absolute worst. I had just finished my fourth of eight cycles of chemo, and had already lost all of my hair. We went to dinner and a play, and as we were leaving the theatre, a horse-drawn carriage was waiting for us outside. He said that he wasn't proposing because he thought my time was limited, but rather to give me something to live for. It was the most wonderful thing that could have uplifted my spirits."
Katie Mandra; diagnosed in 1998 at the age of 22; housewife

"A long-time male friend sent me an e-mail during my treatment that moved me deeply. It still does. He wrote, 'I should really tell you that when times get rough for me, I find the courage and strength I need from the examples set by a handful of people I think of as heroes – one of whom, for a long time, has been you.' As a friend and confidant he was there during two years of breast cancer hell – by phone, by e-mail or over Kung Pao chicken at the local Chinese restaurant."
Alysa Cummings; diagnosed in 1998 at the age of 45; educational trainer

"My male friends have been very supportive and are always ready with a compliment to boost my spirits. They're also ready to join me for a spur-of-the-moment dinner out. When my hair started falling out, a very good male friend shaved my head. We didn't intend it, but it was a slightly erotic experience. Later, I ran into an ex-lover whom I hadn't seen in a while. He still wanted to sleep with me, even after hearing that I'd had a mastectomy. He told me flat out that it didn't matter. While I wasn't ready physically or emotionally for a sexual encounter, he made me feel desirable in a way that I hadn't felt for a long time."

Carrie Drake; diagnosed in 1998 at the age of 42; administrative assistant

"There is life after breast cancer and divorce, because there are many wonderful men out there. I've been out with two of them. The first was Jack. After a few weeks, I told him there was something he should know. He said, 'I think I know what you want to tell me. I heard long ago that you had breast cancer. I don't care if you have one breast or no breasts, I love you just the way you are!' The second man, Ted, was tougher, because he'd lost his wife to breast cancer. One day, several weeks after we met, he came upstairs thinking I was already dressed. I was in my bra, and when he said, 'Oops,' I said, 'I'm glad you are here, because I have to tell you that I had breast cancer 18 years ago.' His response was, 'So what? Is that all you had to tell me? So what do you want to do tonight?' When my divorce is final, Ted and I are going to be married. My children adore him and have learned a great deal from this very caring and loving man. He loves my body, and for the first time in my life I feel special and cherished. Most of all, he loves me."

Miriam Cooper; diagnosed in 1982 at the age of 36; housewife, mother, volunteer, estate agent

"When men you don't know look you over and linger at your breasts even after your surgery, that makes you feel feminine! It was the same thing when a neighbour said he'd take me, no matter what. That made me feel good about myself. I found out how much my husband loved me and how much I was loved for being me, no matter what. My husband has since died and I have a new romantic companion who is fine with the idea that I have only one breast."

Irene Louise; diagnosed in 1995 at the age of 41; retired PA

"I didn't miss one day of work after my surgery – until the day I retired to get married! I had seen Leonard for the first time in 30 years at the wedding of a mutual friend. He had been widowed for two years. When I realised that he was romantically inclined towards me, I made him look at one side of my chest. I watched closely and he didn't wince, just expressed sympathy at what I'd had to undergo. We got married in 1994 and have lived happily ever after."

Lorraine J. Pakkala-Lintala; diagnosed in 1992 at the age of 62; editor, author

"After my divorce, an old friend – male – came back into my life. During my bout with breast cancer, he held me, nurtured me and made me feel feminine and desirable. It was just what I needed. He didn't care about my scars. So I went on to conquer other problems. I had a total knee replacement just after my radiotherapy was finished, and now I can walk with no pain and know that I am cancer-free at the same time. It's a lot to celebrate, and celebrate I do."

Judy Komitee; diagnosed in 1998 at the age of 52; secretary

Last But Not Least

"Consider what it is like to be a man with breast cancer. When I went to a renowned hospital and was directed to the proper department, my daughter, a nurse, and I had a great laugh at the questionnaire I was given to fill out. After the normal name and such, I was asked the following: When did I start my last period? How often did I have it? Was it regular? How many times had I been pregnant? Have I gone through the menopause? Somehow these questions did not fit the patient. The final laugh was when the nurse came out and called for Miss Browne, and my daughter had to point to me as the patient. The good news was that I was told to start thinking years rather than months."

Gerald Browne; diagnosed in 1995

13 · Exercise

Making the Body Better

've always believed in physical exercise. It has been a stress reliever for me since way back when I was a full-time mother with three young, curious, mischievous, conspiratorial and tirelessly athletic boys at home. I spent years as a swimmer, followed by years as a walker. Then I got breast cancer and, after surgery, found myself with limited mobility in my arms and with chest muscles that were good for nothing. My doctors had given me exercises with the instructions that I should start them immediately, but I had barely recovered from the surgery when I began the saline expansion phase of my reconstruction. Exercise? Are you kidding? I hurt too much for that.

So, ignoring those who warned of permanent disability if I didn't start moving asap, I waited until my permanent implants were in and the incision had healed, then began doing exercise videos at home. The videos were basic and didn't take more than 30 minutes on any given day, but they were gentle enough to be fun. Over the next few months I did them four to five times a week — and lo and behold, with barely any pain, I gradually regained full mobility of my arms. My chest wall settled and grew stronger, so that I was able to carry home shopping from the supermarket again. But those exercise videos made other things happen, too. My shoulders became broad and my hips narrow. My back grew more flexible and my legs stronger. In short, my post-cancer body became *better* than the body I'd had before!

With this in mind, I knew from the start that I wanted to have a chapter in *UPLIFT* on the merits of physical exercise following breast cancer treatment. Then, last October, I heard about the women who were rowing in a regatta wearing pink spandex oufits and sparkly baseball caps. All were breast cancer survivors – eight rowers, plus a coxswain – propelling the aptly named *One in Nine* boat in the premier rowing event of the year.

I was familiar with rowing. Two of my sons had rowed at university. I knew about the weight watching and body building that preceded a race, and the bloodied hands and extreme exhaustion that followed. I knew how much of a team effort rowing was – and how positively, utterly gruelling it was. I also knew that the chest and upper arms were major players in the sport. I couldn't begin to imagine women who'd had breast surgery being able to row. Yet there they were, fully competitive.

It took me a while before I was able to get a name and number, but no time at all after that before Diane Cotting, the boat's organiser and a crew member, and Holly Metcalf, the boat's coach, were in my kitchen. While Diane gave me the history of the *One in Nine* boat, a profile of its members, and a taste of its spirit, Holly explained the mechanics – the theory that after extensive breast surgery, it is necessary to re-educate the muscles, to reconfigure them, so that they work in different ways to achieve the same, if not better, results.

That theory made sense to me. Wasn't I spending my summers kayaking, using my arms and shoulders in ways that would have been remarkable even without my having had breast cancer? Granted, I had no desire to row as these women defined it. But if they inspired me, I knew they would inspire others. With Diane's help, I contacted other members of the team. I wanted to know how and why they rowed.

"I started rowing when I was 46," Nancy Oken said. "I was 53 and at the top of my form when I got breast cancer. Afterwards, I decided that I was not going to reverse the personal strides I had made through my rowing. I rowed in a national competition in a boat that won a silver medal. I also rowed in a double with another woman who'd had breast cancer. We wanted to prove to ourselves that we were up to the same challenges as the rest of the rowers."

Like Nancy, Diane had rowed before having breast cancer. She had formed strong friendships with her teammates, and those women were her major support group when she was diagnosed. "They called in all their contacts to make sure I was with the best caregivers in the world. But I never stopped thinking of rowing. It was my lifeline to health and personal sanity. I explained this to each of my doctors. They told me they would do everything in their power to get me back on the water."

Beth Meister had never rowed before. She had watched her daughter row, though, and started rowing as a way to control how she looked – "I wanted to be solid and not jiggly" – when her oncologist put her on Tamoxifen and predicted she would gain weight. Pat Carr started rowing more as a factor of age than of breast cancer. "I was thinking, 'If not now, when?' Besides, I wanted to find out if I could do it." And Mary Ruddell, who didn't start rowing until two or three years after having breast cancer, said, "No one told me that I couldn't do it – but then, I didn't ask."

These women faced obstacles. But they were determined. "When I first went back to rowing, I felt so weak," said Michele Marks, "but I knew that my strength would come back with hard work." Beth had a problem with numbness in her left arm and hand. "So I chose to row port, which meant that I didn't have to 'feather' (turn the oar blade) with that hand." For Mary, the answer was yoga. "Once I had stretched out the scar tissue with yoga, I was ready to go!" Diane had had TRAM-flap reconstruction. That meant her stomach muscles were displaced, which spelled an even greater adjustment. "My plastic surgeon was afraid that I wouldn't be able to do the sit-up motion necessary for a strong stroke. He made me promise that I wouldn't do any abdominal work for six months, and I kept my word. Then, when I started physiotherapy, no one seemed to understand the nature of my reconstruction. I finally started working with a personal trainer, who taught me how to strengthen other muscle groups to replace the muscles I was missing. I learned how to support my body in new ways, so that I would be able to do the motions necessary to pull hard and row well in a boat."

I asked about setbacks. Other than a passing remark from one about causing strain by overcompensating, and from another about once pulling a muscle, none of the women responded. They did respond, though, when I asked about the rewards.

"Rowing brought my self-confidence back," Joyce Abercrombie said. "Whether physical or psychological or both, the benefits were real. Continuing to row after having breast cancer helped me to focus on maintaining a normal life, rather than focusing on the disease." Michele elaborated, "When I'm rowing, all I have to think about is rowing. Nothing else. It is such a relief and release. Same with knowing I have the support of the other women, and knowing I am not alone."

"Rowing gives me a wonderful feeling of strength," said Pat. Mary added, "In season, I'm on the water three or four days a week. Rowing allows you to feel alive and one with the Earth and your soul." Beth summed up both thoughts: "Rowing is good for fitness, strength and endurance – not to mention an appreciation of the beauty of the river."

So what, specifically, of the *One in Nine* boat experience? I asked.

"The *One in Nine* boat has given me an opportunity to revisit my trauma and renew all that is positive," said Beth. "It enables me to show other women that breast cancer is just another challenge. I'll never forget meeting the other women in the boat for the first time, feeling the positive energy and seeing the brilliance of their smiles. These things told me that we did indeed share something. We bonded easily. For most of us, it was the first opportunity we had to openly discuss our experiences."

For Pat, rowing in the *One in Nine* boat meant going public. "Only now, four years later, do people in the club where I regularly row know that I had breast cancer, and that is due to my participation in this boat and the publicity that accompanied it. I never wanted to 'use' breast cancer as an excuse when I was with coaches or fellow rowers."

Not that the women of the *One in Nine* boat rowed silently. When one wears pink spandex tops and glittery baseball caps, one doesn't have to say a word, and people hear. "The day we got our uniforms for the race was funny," Michele recalled. "We went to try on our tops, and they were all so small that we could see every dent, dimple, and scar. We could also see when one breast was larger than the other. We all commented on that."

Beth had her own thoughts on that uniform. "I like to think of myself as a serious rower. Rowing in the *One in Nine* boat challenged that image. We were given hot-pink-and-black skintight outfits and pink sequinned caps to wear in the race. This was good, because everyone could spot us and cheer. But someone took a picture of me from the top of one of the bridges as we rowed underneath, and it appeared on the cover of a rowing magazine. There was no story, just the 'cover girl' picture. To my horror – though I have no *idea* why I left the house that way that day – I was wearing full jewellery in the race!"

Then she ended with a story that gave me goose pimples. "The *One in Nine* boat was rowing up to the start in the regatta. We were getting more excited and anxious as we saw the other boats full of powerful-looking women who would be our competition. Typically, at the start of a race, crews try to scare and demoralise the other crews by looking big and mean. So I was prepared for a cold and threatening reception from these competitors. Instead, as we approached, they began beating the sides of their boats with their palms, unified in a rousing cheer for us – '*One in Nine, One in Nine, One in Nine.*' It was an incredible once-in-a-lifetime reception at the start of a regatta!"

Comparing myself with these women, I feel puny. Lest you feel the same, let me bring the rowing experience down to our level by going back a bit. Believe it or not, it wasn't so very long ago that Diane was actually afraid to start rowing again. "My friends were protective after my surgery, trying to ease me back on to the water without putting pressure on me. So one friend told a little fib. She said that her back was sore and she was too nervous to take a single shell out by herself. She asked me to join her in a double to take the strain off her, in case she ran into trouble. I was paddling away in no time. The feeling was fantastic."

So there. You and I can paddle. Piece of cake.

In the Beginning

"Start walking. Put on an oversized top and just do it. You are sure to feel better when you get moving."
Linda Dyer; diagnosed in 1993 at the age of 40; magazine editor

"Walk every day – even if it's only a short walk. This is great for everything!"
Debbie MacLean; diagnosed in 1991 at the age of 47; volunteer, hospital gift shop and hospice

"Keep at it. Take it slowly, but keep doing it. It will get better, and you will feel better for doing it."
Mary Ruddell; diagnosed in 1992 at the age of 44; programme manager

"The best exercise for mobility: walking my fingers up the shower wall. I felt great excitement each time I climbed another tile!"
Barbara Jentis; diagnosed in 1983 at the age of 41; lawyer

"Years ago, my daughter gave me a little blue Smurf. When I was doing exercises in bed, I would put him on the headboard. My goal was to touch his nose. I finally did! That arm is stronger today than the other arm!"
Barbara C. Sumner; diagnosed in 1982 at the age of 59; housewife

"After my surgery, my husband tied ropes around door knobs, set up pulleys and cut up newspapers for me to scrunch up and throw into a wastepaper basket."
Irene Louise; diagnosed in 1995 at the age of 41; retired PA

"I had trouble getting full mobility back in my arm. I actually had pain that came from not using it enough. I was treating it like a useless appendage. My physiotherapist said to me, 'It's *your* arm!' Such a simple sentence, but it helped me to remember that."
Judith Ormond; diagnosed in 1996 at the age of 49; symphony musician – piccolo

Because You're Worth It!

"When I returned to the fitness centre, I received special attention. I worked with the fitness instructor on a new programme to build myself back up and begin a new healing process."
Sharon Erbe; diagnosed in 1999 at the age of 54; nursing teacher

"Control of my body became an issue. I exercised a lot, cycling and running four miles a day, and I learned an incredible amount about nutrition, particularly antioxidants."
Judith Ormond; diagnosed in 1996 at the age of 49; symphony musician – piccolo

"I was diagnosed at 40 and am a six-year survivor of breast cancer.

One titbit I would like to offer new patients is to start lifting
weights as soon as their doctor allows it. I was not told to do this,
and did not realise the benefits as far as building muscle and gain-
ing better use of the arm after a mastectomy."
Fran DiBiase; diagnosed in 1994 at the age of 40; part-time teacher, part-
time property management executive

"It took me a couple months to feel like exercising after my bilateral mastectomy, but when I did get back to the gym and to a consistent exercise programme, it was the best thing I could have
done! It made me feel healthy and alive. I started cooking and eating healthily, and I felt, for the first time in my life, that I was taking
control and doing something really positive for my body. After
being diagnosed with cancer and feeling very out of control, it was
wonderful to take charge. A healthy diet and regular exercise –
they're good for the body and even better for the mind!"
Julie Crandall; diagnosed in 1998 at the age of 31; housewife and mother

"Work out in ways you didn't before. My upper body is now
stronger than it ever was."
Mindy Greenside; diagnosed in 2000 at the age of 48; midwife

"After my surgery, I took up walking daily with my neighbour for
exercise and also to relieve stress. We still continue this activity. It is
the cheapest therapy I know."
Wanda Null; diagnosed in 1986 at the age of 41; librarian

"Try to get out and walk for some exercise, if you find yourself not
doing any during treatment. Try walking inside a shopping centre
when the weather is bad."
Mary Raffol; diagnosed in 1998 at the age of 44; teacher

"I continued to play tennis between chemo treatments. I had to
stop during radiotherapy because my skin was sensitive, but I
began it again about three weeks after the radiotherapy ended,
when my skin began to heal."
Cornelia Doherty; diagnosed in 1985 at the age of 45; mother, widow,
speaker

"I was so excited when I was able to complete a 3.5-mile sponsored

walk. I was two-thirds of the way through my chemo and couldn't believe how great I felt."
Linda Jones Burns; diagnosed in 2000 at the age of 40; school registrar

"I am a very active, athletic and energetic individual. For the past three years, a group of us have participated in an annual 5km run/walk. I like to race to win and have won in my division the past two years. One big reason for this . . . is the fact that I enter in the survivor category. I stack the odds, so to speak!"
Kathy Kirkley; diagnosed in 1993 at the age of 40; nurse, mother, wife

"As I recuperated I thought about the things that I wanted to do when I was back on my feet and decided that I wanted to run a marathon. Well, it took me seven years and two attempts to do it, but I did complete my first marathon in 1999."
Mary Ruddell; diagnosed in 1992 at the age of 44; programme manager

Go for It!

"Nine months after my breast cancer diagnosis, I realised I was going to live. It was time to rebuild my life. I heard another breast cancer survivor speak of her very positive experience doing yoga, and I decided to give it a try. Timidly, I arranged for one private lesson with her very patient and wise instructor. In that first lesson, I learned that I could control my breath, that my worries disappeared while focusing on gentle stretching and the peace of meditation during savasana. I had a few more private lessons and then tentatively agreed to partner another breast cancer survivor for further lessons. Together we began to learn how to live in the moment, to breathe into the stiffness for more stretch, to concentrate to hold poses, and the joy and healing of deep relaxation. I realised that I did have some control over my body. My arm mobility improved. A friendship developed. Months later, a third breast cancer survivor joined our group. A fourth has now been invited. Yoga on Friday evenings is one of the highlights of my week. I am more at peace with my post-surgical body. Despite the fact that breast cancer is what brought our group together, breast cancer does not exist during that weekly hour."
Sandy Gabriel; diagnosed in 1999 at the age of 45; medical physicist

"About a year after my operation, I started taking yoga lessons. The classes were great, as I was able to stretch various muscles and move in gentle ways that I had not been able to before. It was very freeing to be able to move in ways I had not moved in over a year."

Mary Ruddell; diagnosed in 1992 at the age of 44; programme manager

"I was having trouble getting mobility back in my arm after the mastectomy. I began yoga and swimming. At first I could barely make it across the pool. Now I can swim a mile easily and it feels wonderful."

Diane Wilkinson-Codon; diagnosed in 1999 at the age of 53; massage therapist, nurse

"Only a few short weeks after surgery, I was back in the pool swimming. The mastectomy swimming costume that a friend told me about is not necessary. My chest looks normal in an ordinary swimsuit with a shoulder pad sewn in one side."

Marcia Gibbons; diagnosed in 1991 at the age of 52; artist

"Where I live there are 46 high peaks that hikers climb. My friend did this while undergoing her treatment for breast cancer. It gave her a challenge and the hope that she could beat this disease, and she has!"

Stephanie King; friend of two survivors

"I like to go hiking. During the time when I wasn't strong enough to do that, I tried to take little walks, extending the length of the walk a bit each trip. It was good just to be outdoors, enjoying the sights, sounds and smells of my surroundings, which just happen to be awesome."

Carrie Drake; diagnosed in 1998 at the age of 42; administrative assistant

"Before I was diagnosed with the cancer, I had been losing strength, in my legs especially. I was unable to get out of the bath or to get up off the floor, and I had extreme difficulty getting out of a chair or a car. The doctors were puzzled, and I had many tests, but all were normal. After my cancer surgery, I started to regain my strength. I saw a neurologist, and he confirmed it. The weakness could have been from my body fighting the cancer. I have since heard of other people who have also experienced weakness before cancer was diagnosed. We still don't know for sure, but I do know that I am feeling fine now and am quite active. I am a square dancer and have my old stamina back now, so I am able to do a whole weekend of dancing at a festival."

Diana Vise; diagnosed in 2000; civil service, retired

"I had just been awarded my black belt in karate, after three years of hard work, when I was diagnosed with breast cancer. I feel that being in good physical shape definitely helped me get through the treatment. I continued to exercise and walk daily, which helped me bounce back faster after each treatment. Exercise also helped me have some kind of control of my life again. I felt alive and healthy when I worked out. I also play the piano and I continued to work my 40 hours a week during the whole thing. It's a way to heal yourself mentally."

Kathy Rabassa; diagnosed in 1999 at the age of 34; administrative assistant

"Two things helped me a lot, and these had to do with mental attitude and how I felt about myself. First, I continued to work on my treadmill even when I didn't want to, and my reward was feeling proud of myself and giving myself pats on the back. Second, I had someone around who made me smile. During the worst of it, my youngest son brought me little black and white cows to put on the handlebars of my treadmill to keep me company, and he came home every night and made me giggle with new stories of where he worked. He also prodded me to eat and take my medicine, but it was all done with a grin. If attitude is important, then feeling good about yourself and learning to look for the smiles should be at the top of everyone's list of survival tools."

Barbara Hutchinson; diagnosed in 1995 at the age of 62; retired

"I'm getting around to exercise this year as I battle with the aftermath of breast cancer – menopause! Who would guess that oestrogen could be so helpful with so many little things? Ah, well, hot flushes too will end."

Christine Foutris; diagnosed in 1999 at the age of 49; teacher

14 • Religion

Bringing in the Big Guns

When I initially conceived of *UPLIFT*, I had no plans for a chapter on religion. It wasn't that I didn't think religion was a major factor in many people's lives, especially those who were ill – because I knew that it was. But I felt that there were already plenty of other "inspirational" books on the shelves. I wanted *UPLIFT* to contain the kind of practical info and upbeat stories that hadn't yet been published.

So I didn't mention religion in the guidelines. Nor, though, did I discount submissions that mentioned it from inclusion in the book when they did indeed arrive. How could I? The religion–health link has been documented. Studies have found that when anxious people turn to God, their anxiety is reduced, and when their anxiety is reduced, both their immune systems and their cardiovascular systems get a boost. Moreover, *UPLIFT* survivors repeatedly name their church and its members as a very special kind of support group.

The premise of *UPLIFT* is to tell the good stuff. If faith helps a woman make it through breast cancer with a smile on her face and makes her palm's lifeline longer than ever, those submissions fit the guidelines to a 'T'.

Here they are, short and sweet. Enjoy.

Having Faith

"The most settling thing I did after hearing my diagnosis was to take a walk along the shore of a nearby lake. At one point, I stopped, leaned on a railing overlooking the lake, and looked back at the land. After a while, I simply said, 'God, I don't want to deal with this. I'd like you to handle this one for me. Okay?' That was it, but amazingly then I was able to let go. Not that I didn't do my part in taking very good care of myself, but I never fretted about my diagnosis after that. I just did the next right thing that came along."
Gracie Schwingle; diagnosed in 1998 at the age of 51; secretary

"My daughter left a framed saying next to my bed. It said, 'God is watching you. I know because I asked him to.' "
Corda M. Gilliland; diagnosed in 2000 at the age of 72; retired, widow

"We have a deep faith, and this is what sustained us as a family. We prayed frequently together. I attended daily Mass with my husband as often as I could."
Cornelia Doherty; diagnosed in 1985 at the age of 45; mother, widow, speaker

"The most constructive thing I did after hearing my diagnosis was to have a heart-to-heart talk with God. The most *helpful* thing I did was to learn that one of the members of my church was a ten-year survivor."
Debby Whittet; diagnosed in 1996 at the age of 43; household technician, part-time library worker

"A phone call soon after my diagnosis prompted my involvement in my local religious organisation. The people there were so welcoming that it opened up a whole new world for me with a renewed belief in my faith. This has given me a new and ongoing support system of wonderful people who care about me."
Linda Perkins; diagnosed in 1999 at the age of 35; project manager

"When my mother was diagnosed, I was only 20 and had no idea of the ramifications of it. During two years of surgery and treatments, I encouraged her and celebrated with her when it was finished,

and she is still surviving. Then, when I was expecting my fourth child, my own diagnosis came. It was overwhelming and humbling. What helped me to endure the treatments with four small children? My friends and my church. Being headstrong and independent, I had to learn to receive their kindness. The outpouring of food was so incredible that we had to set up a rota because the refrigerator was overflowing. I was grateful for their generosity, as I certainly didn't feel like cooking. It turned out to be a double blessing. Those who gave were also enriched. I learned that sometimes I am able to do Christ's work by helping others and at other times I am to be helped so that my neighbour can be Christ for me. My faith grew in leaps and bounds! Less than two years later, my sister was diagnosed with cancer. Somehow I couldn't be sad, though I knew how hard her next few months would be. God was working through her as well. I knew that we are survivors. How lucky our family is – and my cancer experience continues to be a blessing. As I work in a pharmacy, many of my patients are receiving the same diagnosis. When I tell them that I have had cancer and am a survivor, it gives them hope."
Jane Zinda; diagnosed in 1987 at the age of 33; mother, pharmacist

"It's not that I ever laughed at people involved in prayer chains, but I was sincerely grateful when they included me."
Kathi Ward; diagnosed in 1994 at the age of 47; promotions executive

"Jeremiah 29:11 has been such a help whenever I begin to doubt. 'For I know the thoughts that I think toward you, saith the Lord, thoughts of peace, and not of evil, to give you a future and a hope.'"
Judy Peterson; diagnosed in 2000 at the age of 58; nurse

"Among my cancer blessings were the 'signs' of love I received from God. For example, for weeks I saw a heart outline on a tarnishing plughole. I'd never seen it before and have never seen it since."
Diane Bongiorno; diagnosed in 1998 at the age of 43; instructional aide

"When I told a dear friend of mine about my diagnosis, she told me about a dove that had been hanging around her house. This dove should have been long gone, since winter was near. But this dove served a purpose. It brought peace somehow to the people who saw it. One day my friend sent me a feather from this dove with a note saying, 'Remember, sometimes God's word rests on the wings of a dove.' It was a sweet reminder of trust in God, and He would give me peace.

"The morning of my mastectomy I was in the shower when I heard my son yelling about a bird in the house. Since we have several caged birds, I assumed one of them had got out. When I got out of the shower, I asked him what all the commotion was about, and he said, 'A bird flew in the house, did one lap of the living room and flew back out.' When I asked him what kind of bird it was, he said it was a white dove. My sister had seen the bird and agreed with that. I knew that God had sent that dove to give me peace and remind me that He is in control. During my recovery and chemotherapy I remembered the dove, God's promise, and my favourite verse, from Proverbs 3:5 and 6: 'Trust in the Lord with all your heart and lean not on your own understanding; in all your ways acknowledge Him and He will make your paths straight.' "
Tammy Delin; diagnosed in 1997 at the age of 33; teacher's assistant

"My friend Alice hated going for her radiotherapy. The lying still really got to her. She finally discovered that if she said the 23rd Psalm, she knew exactly how many times to say it and where she would be when it was over. When I passed this hint on to another good friend, June came out after her treatment one morning with a smile on her face. 'It works,' she said. If you don't know the 23rd Psalm, sing your favourite song to yourself. That works, too!"
Donna Palmer; friend of a survivor

"To strengthen my belief in God, in myself and in life during the chemo, I read an uplifting perpetual calendar verse and psalm daily – and still do."
Sue Braun; diagnosed in 1988 at the age of 41; housewife

"I was given a prayer that I said before each treatment, and it comforted me then and still comforts me now: 'The light of God surrounds me. The love of God enfolds me. The power of God protects me. The presence of God watches over me. Whatever I am, God is, and all is well.' "
Christine Foutris; diagnosed in 1999 at the age of 49; teacher

"I awoke one morning realising that I had entered into another part of my grieving process. I was sad to be losing a part of my body, but I visualised our Lord on the cross, and I thought of the pain that he must have suffered. He did so much for me. I could do this."
Sandy Williams; diagnosed in 1999 at the age of 51; children's public librarian

"Life is a series of choices. My friend Sheryl sent me a story about a carrot, an egg and a coffee bean. The story went like this: 'When you get into hot water, you can choose to be a carrot, an egg or a coffee bean. A carrot becomes soft and pliable, giving in to the adversity, giving up. The egg hardens and refuses to conform. The coffee bean, however, turns the water into a steaming drink full of flavour.' 'You,' Sheryl wrote to me, 'chose to make coffee.' In the past, when my husband or children or close friends have been ill, I have actually prayed to God to give me the illness, to let me carry it. When I knew that I might be facing cancer, I felt God telling me, 'Now's your chance to make coffee.' "
Rosamary Amiet; diagnosed in 2000 at the age of 48; programme manager

"I owe my survival to the Lord Jesus Christ. Every time I go for radiotherapy, I surround myself with prayer. I pray right through the treatment."
Jennie Isbell; diagnosed in 1999 at the age of 76; retired, housewife

"The thing that helped me get through this the most was my faith in God. I have never prayed so hard in all my life. I put everything in God's hands, and asked Him to help me."
Paula Porter; diagnosed in 2000 at the age of 47; telephone operator

"How to deal with the worry? That was a hard one, because two years after my diagnosis, there was another lump. So I turned to God. I had been floating. He grounded me once more. I got the news that it was nothing, but I want to stay grounded. I can face anything laid before me . . . with God."
Pam Waddell; diagnosed in 1998 at the age of 38; writer, teacher's assistant

"This Buddhist prayer helps me to begin each day: 'May all be

loved. May all be healed. May all be sheltered. May all be free from
fear. May I be loved. May I be healed. May I be sheltered. May I be
free from fear.' "
Deb Haney; diagnosed in 1996 at the age of 48; administrative assistant,
artist

"Cancer, for me, was an agenda, giving me permission to live the
way I had been living for years, by faith. God has blessed me with
12 years of survival and many wonderful friends, fellow cancer survivors and their families!"
Aileen Pandapas; diagnosed in 1989 at the age of 41; mother, volunteer,
former secretary

"Looking back, I realise that I have a greater appreciation for the
joys of life, a calmness I never had before, and a deeper faith in
God. What more could I ask?"
E. Mary Lou Clauss; diagnosed in 1991 at the age of 55; retired nurse

"Today is 8th June, 2000. You ask what is so special about this day?
Well, let me tell you, God has blessed me with 19 cancer-free years!
I thought of many ways to celebrate this day, and finally decided to
do a sponsored walk for cancer. Thank you, Lord, for once more
blessing my steps. I can't wait for next year!"
Debbie Roberts; diagnosed in 1981 at the age of 22; housewife, mother

"Someone wrote, 'Having cancer was the best thing that ever happened to me.' Originally, I thought this was a stupid statement. I
could not comprehend how anyone could say this. But, after the
past year, I agree. My wife having cancer was the best thing that
ever happened to us. In looking back, I was a religious snob. I felt
that going to church weekly, saying my daily prayers and occasionally volunteering for our parish kept me in touch with God and
my salvation. But I stopped going through the motions when
Joanne was diagnosed with breast cancer. I started to pray with my
heart. I found prayer an answer to life's problems. Had it not
been for my wife's cancer, I would have never reached this level of
understanding."
Gene Palmer; Joanne's husband

"We named my cancer Jack. During the weekly trips to hospital with my husband, *Hit the Road, Jack* and *You Are My Sunshine* became our theme songs. Jack did indeed hit the road. Prayer was powerful."

Joanne Palmer; diagnosed in 1996 at the age of 42; medical receptionist

15 • Pure Uplift

Wrapping It Up with a Bow

So we've discussed specifics, like hair, food and clothes. We've talked about what we want, how we feel and what others can do to help. We've gone through tactics for regaining control. We've done the positive attitude thing. What's left? Nothing but wrapping it up.

This chapter is for miscellaneous thoughts that might just as easily have fitted into several other chapters but didn't instantly slip into any one. We're talking about some wonderful bits of philosophy here, like that from Rosamary Amiet, who wrote, "My single most important piece of advice for a friend is, don't spend time worrying how to live with breast cancer. Spend your time learning how to live life." And that from Sallie Burdine, who wanted to pass on something she'd read: "Attitude is the mind's paintbrush. It can colour any situation." And from Betsy Ellis Bowles, who wrote, "We do have *some* control over the length of our life, but the real kick comes from knowing that we have *much* control over its width and depth. If we're not doing what makes our hearts sing, we're wasting precious time."

And then, there are a few special anecdotes, like this one sent in by Darlene Jurow: "My breast reconstruction involved using stomach tissue to form two new breasts. Due to the incision from hip to hip, I had trouble standing up straight for several months. Upon seeing my distress, my husband ran out and bought me three antique canes. One had a built-in flask . . . a wee nip for the times when the pain was gripping. One had a concealed dagger to poke those who jokingly called me an old crone (I was only 52). The last had a compass in the handle to direct me back to my family. These three treasures have been my 'support'. They represent comfort, self-esteem and love. Internal strength comes in strange packages!"

Not so strange a package, by now, is *UPLIFT*. You may already be well versed in the attitude, but a little more never hurts. Read and reread. As so many survivors say, "If it feels good, do it!"

So Much to Appreciate

"Breast cancer has helped me not to take anything for granted. I'm content with even the smallest of things, like doing cross-stitch, having time to read, visiting my family and friends, or watching my cats play and sleep. These are all special moments."
Gwen Loverink; diagnosed in 1994 at the age of 34; police dispatcher

"I was 36 years old and six months pregnant when I was diagnosed, and had a mastectomy and chemo treatments during my pregnancy. I certainly never expected this at a time that should have been so happy, but we are certainly happy now. My child and I are both survivors!"
Tammi Keller; diagnosed in 2000 at the age of 36; mother

"My sister and several of my friends have had breast cancer, and all are doing well. When I was diagnosed, I told myself that if they got through it, so would I. Now, after 33 radiotherapy sessions, I am a survivor, too. The key to success, I think, is a positive attitude and a good outlook."
Ellie Meyers; diagnosed in 2000 at the age of 70; retired civil servant

"I will never forget the feeling of warmth and caring I received when a total stranger approached me in a department store at the time when my 'chemo hair' was just starting to grow. She had the courage to ask me if I had undergone chemotherapy and was it for breast cancer. When I answered yes, she gave me the longest, hardest hug of encouragement, and I nearly cried. She had a daughter who was a recent survivor, and she wanted to pass on the feeling

that 'You can do it, too.' This unknown woman has made me want
to be just as courageous and pass on the needed hugs, so my eyes
and ears are always open. I am very proud to be recognised as a survivor and never want to lose that image, so I am keeping my hair
short and wispy as a sign to everyone."
Sarah Stuart; diagnosed in 1999 at the age of 52; banking personnel
assistant

"A positive attitude makes such a difference. It is a fact that it
affects survivor rates in cancer patients. Quality of life is also
improved by a positive attitude. How to stay positive? Take one day
at a time and deal with each problem as it comes. Don't let your
mind anticipate new ones. They might never occur."
Judy Peterson; diagnosed in 2000 at the age of 58; nurse

"How is my post-cancer body better? Physically, I'm a bit leaner,
so I feel better about my shape and weight. Mentally – more
importantly – I appreciate so much more, each and every
moment that makes up the day. *And* I no longer tolerate rude or
narrow-minded people!"
Carrie Drake; diagnosed in 1998 at the age of 42; administrative assistant

"I've always felt grateful for the wonderful people and things in my
life, and I continue to do so. Whether my appreciation of these
things is part of growing older, or getting cancer, or what, I don't
know. I sincerely hope that my compassion, volunteering, fundraising or whatever small part I can play will help someone else
with breast cancer."
Sheila Roper; diagnosed in 1995 at the age of 57; housewife

"Now, at the dinner table, each member of our family says what we
are grateful for. It doesn't have to be a serious thing – it may be
football – just as long as we are all appreciating the abundance in
our lives. We are all so blessed. Let us pay attention to what is right
instead of what is wrong."
Sandy Rodgers; diagnosed in 1999 at the age of 44; mother, nurse, Reiki
master

"I ate well during chemo in order to keep my blood counts as high
as possible. I cried when I had to and smiled the rest of the time. I

counted the days when chemo was over and then breezed through radiotherapy. I kept saying over and over, 'This too shall pass.' Now, when annoying little things happen, I compare them to that time in my life, and it puts everything in perspective. This Christmas was wonderful. I enjoyed every moment and never complained. I plan to enjoy many more!"

Frances Gallello; diagnosed in 2000 at the age of 51; mental health assistant

"You know that saying about taking time to smell the roses? Nothing could be more true, especially for those of us who've had breast cancer. I've just been to Paris with three friends, and I don't work Saturdays now or let myself get stressed out the way I used to. I've just bought myself a car I've always wanted. It is gorgeous and I love love love driving it!"

Patti R. Martinez; diagnosed in 1999 at the age of 54; estate agent

"I was diagnosed a year and a half ago and had a lumpectomy and radiotherapy. Having been an oncology nurse for several years, I must say that it was both frightening and enlightening to have the boot on *my* foot! My breast cancer was discovered though a routine mammogram, as so many are, and my experience was a positive one."

Donna Barnett; diagnosed in 1999 at the age of 40; nurse

"My mother is grateful for the benefits and blessings she has received regarding her bout with breast cancer. She believes that breast cancer survivors, those currently undergoing treatment for breast cancer and those whose lives have most recently been turned upside down because of a mysterious lump are truly a sisterhood whose collective motto includes strength, determination, optimism, love and prayer."

John E. Schlimm II; son of survivor Barbara Schlimm

"Never ask yourself 'Why me?' It's not only a waste of time and energy, it's a misconception. Look around you at those less fortunate. The world is full of victims – wonderful people who have had bad things happen to them, too. Be faithful, thankful, grateful and keep an open mind. You never know what tomorrow will bring, and it just might be a cure."

Kathy Weaver-Stark; diagnosed in 1991 at the age of 46; loss adjuster, instructor

Every Day Is a Gift

"I am a seven-and-a-half-year breast cancer survivor whose disease was diagnosed during my eighth month of pregnancy. Now, as I take part in a sponsored walk for cancer every September with my beautiful daughter Eve (Hebrew for 'life'), who wears a sign on her back that says 'In celebration of my mama', I realise that God presented me with a challenge, but he also gave me a great gift."
Renee C. Johannesen; diagnosed in 1993 at the age of 35; marketing communications manager

"It has been seven years since my diagnosis, and I live life as fully as I can. Whenever I hesitate to do something I'm too tired to do, I push myself. I thank God every day for this strength and for giving me another day."
Alyce Feinstein; diagnosed in 1993 at the age of 58; administrative assistant

"I am a very lucky 42-year-old married woman with three sons aged 16, 13, and nine. I believe that we are given this 'gift' of illness to see how special and fragile life is. The gift may not be wanted, but it can teach a most valuable lesson: to love and live fully in our day-to-day lives."
Cathy Hanlon; diagnosed in 2000 at the age of 42; school researcher

"Say to yourself daily, 'I can beat this.' A positive attitude will give you the courage to go on when things get rough. Most important, remember that you are not alone!"
Cheryl Cavallo; diagnosed in 1997 at the age of 35; housewife

"My treatment began in the autumn, during the football season. Our son, Jay, played football and we had tried not to miss any of his matches. As the weather got colder, though, my doctor warned me about staying well and told me – absolutely – not to attend the next football match. I explained to our son that I wouldn't be able to attend and he said that he understood and that he just wanted me to be well. Later I got a call from the football coach, who had seen that Jay and his friends were down, and was worried that if I wasn't there, they might not be able to concentrate on the game. Then he asked to speak to my husband.

"My husband hung up the phone, bundled me up in my coat, boots, hat and gloves, and off we went. When we arrived at the ground, we were taken to the section reserved for the media. In this booth, they had a cosy chair for me with an electric heater at my feet and a nice blanket just in case I needed it. The coach came in and asked whether I was comfortable, and then asked me to do him a favour. He asked me to watch him on the pitch during the warm up, and to stand up when he waved to me. He left and went on to the pitch and called the players together. He then waved to me, and I responded by standing and gave a wave of my own. The boys saw me in the booth, pointed to our position and began clapping Jay on the back. It seems that our son had told his friends that I wouldn't be able to attend the game. I believe he did understand but was still worried about his mum, which in turn worried the other boys. Two of his good friends had gone to ask the coach to check up on me and he decided that they wouldn't believe I was truly well unless they saw me. I can't tell you who won that football match, but I can tell you how uplifted I was by the show of love and kindness, not only for me, but for our son as well."

Brenda Carr; diagnosed in 1988 at the age of 40; wife, mother, retired school counsellor

"When I see my tattoo marks from radiotherapy or my lack of a breast and begin to feel sorry for myself, I stop short and remember that since my diagnosis I have seen my son marry and my daughter leave school and go off to college. Every day is a gift."

Joanne Tutschek; diagnosed in 1988 at the age of 55; research communications director

When I Grow Up

"I don't recommend getting breast cancer as a way of helping you decide what you want to be when you grow up, but for me, the diagnosis and subsequent mastectomy and chemotherapy were the wake-up call that helped convince me to abandon a gruelling one-hour-each-way commute to a windowless office for a job closer to home. I had always wanted to be a novelist and as I faced my own mortality I thought, '*If not now, when?*' Eighteen years later, I am the author of three published novels (whose heroine is

a breast cancer survivor), one collaborative novel (with 12 other women), and a lot of short stories."
Marcia Talley; diagnosed in 1983 at the age of 39; mystery novelist

"Getting my diagnosis in 1992 gave me the courage to pursue my lifelong dream of becoming a nurse. I felt that if I could beat cancer, I could do this. Going back into education at the age of 39 was great for my self-esteem. I found that I was able to talk to the younger women about the importance of examining your own breasts. I calmed their fears. They told me that I was an inspiration to them and their mothers, because I had a zest for life. Well, I'd been able to get rid of all the negative things in my life. For me, life truly began after breast cancer."
Deborah Parker; diagnosed in 1991 at the age of 34; nurse

"After I was diagnosed with breast cancer, my realisation that I was not, after all, immortal led me to focus on what I have long believed is the one thing that I have a responsibility for improving: education. That was more than eight years ago, and I am still doing everything in my power to see that education in general, and the teaching of reading and writing in particular, improves."
Annelle Houk; diagnosed in 1988 at the age of 59; writer, editor

"I took a course offered by the hospital that pointed out the importance of a positive outlook. This was not an easy course, because it talked about giving yourself time for things like meditation and paying attention to your own needs. It didn't tell you how to start doing this after spending 47 years without. Around this same time, I was told of a woman psychotherapist who specialised in treating cancer patients. I went on to have many sessions with her, concentrating on cleaning old hurts and grievances out of my psyche. Then I radically changed my life. Among other things, I moved to a big city for an academic year, going back to the art I enjoyed when I was younger. During this time, I learned to see myself separately from my family, and, as a result, could cope much better with everything. The best part is that I am now an emerging artist."
Carol Pasternak; diagnosed in 1986 at the age of 47; artist

"What have I done in between chemo and radiotherapy? I started oil painting again after 15 years. And I've started an afghan. I haven't made one in years. The one thing I'm really proud of is that I'm going to open my own business in two months. I saw a great need for a wig shop in this area. Having had cancer, I understand the importance of looking good as you go through treatment. Everything has fallen into place for the shop, which tells me this was meant to be. The landlord is supporting me all the way. We have lots of renovating to do, but my boyfriend is a jack-of-all-trades and the few people who know of my plan have volunteered to help! Who could ask for more?"

Sharon Daniels; diagnosed in 2000 at the age of 49; hairdresser, wig shop owner

Longevity

"At 34, I thought I was too young for cancer. But I wasn't. I had an eight-year-old daughter and a budding career and no time for something like this. The hardest part was the seven months of chemo. I figured that if I could survive the cure, I'd be fine. I'm proud to be approaching my 20th anniversary and am a huge proponent of self-examinations and regular check-ups. Women owe it to themselves!"

Marti Devich; diagnosed in 1980 at the age of 34; sales, business owner, writer

"When my radiotherapy ended, I bought a five-year-calendar. I am proud to report that the pages of that calendar are now only a month shy of five full wonderful years. I've just bought another one!

Suzanne Pollock; diagnosed in 1995 at the age of 50; stationer

"Seven years cancer-free is marvellous!"

Alyce Feinstein; diagnosed in 1993 at the age of 58; administrative assistant

"My husband was quite ill when I was diagnosed with breast cancer. I had only been home from hospital for a few days when he died and I had to face the anguish of that. After my incision healed, I had 38 days of radiotherapy and every day I would set off alone to travel eight miles for the treatment. It helped that after each one I would have lunch, go shopping or to see a film. I will be 86 next

birthday and have just moved into a beautiful retirement home.
They take wonderful care of me here. What a life. God has been
good to me."
Dorothy A. Wilson; diagnosed in 1995 at the age of 80; retired

"My mother was a long-time survivor who lived to see her *grandchildren* leave school, get married and have children of their own."
Betty Pollom; daughter of Frances Davis

"It's okay to be afraid. Watch your own body and mind, and tell your
doctors if you feel that something isn't right. Don't be afraid to
speak up for yourself – but don't worry. After a few years, you won't
think every headache is a brain tumour, and breast cancer will *not*
be the first thing you think of when you wake up in the morning."
Eleanor Anbinder; diagnosed in 1991 at the age of 50; sales manager

"I was given the best piece of advice by my oncologist when I raced
in, terrified because I'd found a tiny lump on my leg. 'Yep, it's a
lump,' he said. 'You're going to get lots of lumps and bumps, and
you're entitled to them.' I think every cancer survivor gets in a
panic over every ache, pain, lump or bump for quite a while. Don't
be foolish; get them checked out if they hang around. But they are
no more likely to be cancer than they were before you had your
mastectomy."
Lynne Rutenberg; diagnosed in 1980 at the age of 35; retired teacher

"Aches and pains are a problem. So is growing older. I mean, I'm
only 55, but my body doesn't recover from bruises and sprains as
quickly as it did when I was 20. Add to that the fact that I'm now
into working out and power walking, and you have muscle sprains
and aches that last a while. When to worry? I asked my doctor
about this. She said she would be glad to check out anything that
worried me, if it would put my mind at ease. She also said that as
each year passed, I would become more comfortable with those
aches and pains. She's been right on both counts."
Barbara Delinsky; diagnosed in 1994 at the age of 49; writer

"When I returned home from hospital, it was July. The flowers were
blooming profusely, the grass was pretty and green, the sun was
shining brightly and I marvelled at the beauty of God's Earth,

which I had not appreciated like this before. That was 46 years ago. I have lived to see my grandchildren and great-grandchildren. Since then I have had some of the happiest days of my life."
Willie Mae Ashley; diagnosed in 1954 at the age of 37; writer, retired saleswoman

"My mother had a radical mastectomy during the 1930s. She also had to go the radiotherapy route. Her body was scarred, but she had no recurrence. She lived to be 91!"
Alice Bruneau; daughter of a survivor

"It has been more than eight years since my mastectomy. In that time, my cancer has been transformed from a 'C' to a 'c'. After thinking I'd been given a death sentence, my stubbornness and determination took over. What had been fear and rage now became 'Get out of my way; I have work to do.' I was determined to continue teaching, finish my post-graduate course in special needs education and get back on the tennis courts as soon as possible. But if we want to talk of fearless survivors, I have to talk about the special kids with whom I've worked over the past 13 years. These are kids unable to attend school because of physical and/or emotional problems. My job is to go to their homes every day for one to two hours of tuition. There have been kids with broken legs and kids with emotional problems. Some are stricken with AIDS, sickle cell anemia or cancer. As I struggled to keep working through my treatments, these kids kept me going, telling me to eat well, to get lots of rest and do all the things that make me smile. They would ring my home on treatment days to tell my partner what side effects might occur and how to deal with them. As the years have passed, my concerns have slowly but surely disappeared. With each year, my level of physical and emotional well-being has become stronger and stronger. It's okay that my body is shaped like a pear. I am comfortable with myself. After all, I am here. I am a survivor."
Carol Snyder; diagnosed in 1992 at the age of 47; special needs teacher

"My friend Ruth and her husband Marshall were part of our poker group for nearly 40 years. When Marshall was diagnosed with lymphoma, Ruthie spent the entire time with him, sharing a semi-private room. She went home only to bathe, feed the cat and check the post. Then, one month after Marshall died, after being his

bulwark for nearly five years, Ruthie was diagnosed with breast cancer. Who would be her support? We always teased the Pollocks about the number of children they had – three girls and two boys – a 'full house'. Ruthie tells us that her great 'hand' and their spouses saw her through her mastectomy and reconstruction. Fifteen years have passed since then. Ruthie has travelled all over the country and to many foreign countries. Apart from her travels, she is particularly proud of completing a 55-mile walk for breast cancer awareness, during which she turned 65. What a way to celebrate a birthday and what a woman! She is a role model for us all!"
Rae Shapiro; friend of Ruth Pollock

"The mantra I was given to repeat daily: 'Anything less than growing old is simply not acceptable.'"
Betsy Ellis Bowles; diagnosed in 2000 at the age of 57; private mortgage banker

The Best Thing about Having Breast Cancer

"Breast cancer, like any other illness, is one of life's teachers. What do we take away from it? That depends on each of us. We can't change our situation, but we can make the most of it. We can take time to slow down and really care for ourselves, something that is often hard for women to do. We can also become more compassionate about the suffering of others, and there are plenty of people with worse problems and challenges than ours. We can become more spiritual, more physically healthy, more focused on what is really important in our lives. We can be more thankful for the love that surrounds us."
Deb Haney; diagnosed in 1996 at the age of 48; administrative assistant, artist

"For me, breast cancer was a wake-up call. I worry less about things I have no control over and focus on what is important to me."
Debby Whittet; diagnosed in 1996 at the age of 43; housewife, part-time library worker

"Breast cancer has changed my life in a way that is almost hard to describe. There is no room for negativity in my life now. Everything and everyone are more special to me than ever. I try every

day to recognise my wealth of good family, good friends and good attitude."
Jennifer Wersal; diagnosed in 2000 at the age of 30; marketing executive

"I wouldn't wish breast cancer on my worst enemy, but for me, it was one of the best experiences of my life. It gently moved me along on my spiritual journey and made me stop and rethink priorities."
Sandy Williams; diagnosed in 1999 at the age of 51; children's public librarian

"I have heard some women say that they were thankful for their cancer diagnoses. I wouldn't go that far, but it did make me take stock of my life and decide what was important and what was not. Although I have always been a Christian, I am more spiritual now and, I think, a much better person. My husband Jay and I always talked about buying a big truck and hitting the road when our kids were old enough. We did that the year after my diagnosis. It has been a great experience. We have been over almost all of the country and have enjoyed every minute of it."
Rebecca Clarkson; diagnosed in 1997 at the age of 45; road transport worker

"In less than two years, I experienced breast cancer through my two best friends. It changed all of our lives, because we realised that the silly things in life that we took so seriously before weren't so important after all. The words of the old expression 'When you have your health, you have everything' are the truest words ever written."
Grace Trocco; friend of two survivors

"My best friend was diagnosed nearly two years ago, and what a frightening thing it was! She had two young children who really needed her, along with her family and friends. We fought together, laughed together, and cried together – and she is wonderful today! No more wigs, no more chemotherapy; she is clean! What a joy! It makes all of us appreciate life and love so very much!"
Pat West; friend of a survivor

"I see the world differently now. I don't take life so seriously. Since

being diagnosed, I have travelled to all the places I wanted to see. I'm more spontaneous. I lost my beautiful blonde curly hair and every single hair on my body, but that meant I didn't have to shave or shampoo my hair. It meant that I had a low-maintenance body and could be ready to go anywhere in seconds, instead of hours. I was proud to be bald, because I was alive. I'm not afraid or embarrassed to tell people I love them. I am living with a vengeance."
Cindy Bird; diagnosed in 1998 at the age of 39; personnel officer

"This has been a tough battle, but it's also been one of the most wonderful journeys I've ever taken. I've met the most remarkable people. I've learned that the human spirit is truly alive and well. I can honestly say that I do not regret having breast cancer."
Val Long; diagnosed in 1999 at the age of 47; administrative assistant

"Since having breast cancer, I am less afraid in some ways and more in others. I now ride on roller-coasters and in helicopters, and take physical risks more often, and I feel great about that. I am, however, much more neurotic about every little bump, lump or pain."
Suzanne Pollock; diagnosed in 1995 at the age of 50; stationer

"Going through breast cancer is no piece of cake, but the benefits are endless. I believe that fear is the single most deadly emotion I had to deal with."
Alyce Feinstein; diagnosed in 1993 at the age of 58; administrative assistant

"Only positive things have come out of my having breast cancer. I have learned to enjoy the smallest of life's pleasures. I have learned that nothing is a crisis unless it is fatal. I have learned not to complain about getting up in the morning. My circle of friends has become larger than life – all kinds of friends, all very important to me. I've learned to take time each day to be thankful for what I have, not what I want. I remember that God only gives me what I can handle."
Jacki Anthony; diagnosed in 1998 at the age of 48; nurse

"I learned to let family and friends take care of me. My husband went with me to the first chemo treatment, but after that a different friend accompanied me each time. Friends cleaned my

house, brought food, took me shopping and sent me books. My children 'created' a T-shirt with all their names on it – including a two-year-old handprint and a grand-dog pawprint. Another thing I learned? To let people pray with me and for me. These gestures of love, friendship and faith generate a wonderful sense of well-being."
Faye Hardiman; diagnosed in 1998 at the age of 50; wife, mother, teacher

"Perhaps the most significant outcome of my battle with breast cancer is that I have changed my outlook on life. I now regard life as precious and try not to focus on negative things. Eliminating stress and resentment from my life and concentrating on the positive has become my goal. I am now more at peace with myself."
Sandy Mark; diagnosed in 1998 at the age of 55; administrative assistant

"Breast cancer has taught me to accept what I cannot change, to listen with an open heart and to love myself. It has taught me to look at small wonders; to appreciate sunshine, rain and wind; and to value the love of family and friends. I have a wonderful sister, and our time together is precious to me. At a special time of day, we each light a candle and think of each other."
Nan Comstock; diagnosed in 1988 at the age of 39; self-employed

"Cancer has changed me more than it has changed my life. I have always laughed a lot and I continue to do so. But my soul is deeper and wiser, and I can see the small stuff from the rest. I don't save my china for a special day. Every day is special!"
Dot Heimer; diagnosed in 1999 at the age of 56; certified dental assistant

"It seems weird to say that breast cancer could in any way improve my life, but it has. I am halfway through chemo, and it is rough. But I have found that I am one who has taken my marriage, family and life for granted. My husband is 200 per cent there for me, and I have found so many wonderful qualities in him that I never would have known if it were not for this disease. It's too bad that it took something like this to make me realise what a good life I have."
Lori Bartz; diagnosed in 2000 at the age of 41; customer service representative

"The best thing about breast cancer? I am truly happier now than I was before the diagnosis. My slight fear of recurrence is my friendly reminder to live fully. After every check-up visit, I celebrate. We have a special dinner and I dance around, knowing that I'm healthy. It more than makes up for the nervousness I feel beforehand. Unlike most people, who have check-ups less often, we get the 'good news' of good health every few months. I feel a lightness of being incomparable to anything I felt before cancer."

Sharon Carr; diagnosed in 1997 at the age of 42; hospice grief counsellor

"I was diagnosed in March and operated on in April. Chemo began in June and ended in August. They were six months that totally changed my life and that of my family, but given the option, we would do it all again! Why? I found out that my husband loves me for who I am, not for my breasts. My family was drawn closer together and even closer to God. We do not take any day for granted. And best of all, we've had the opportunity to encourage others in the same situation."

Patti Dempster; diagnosed in 1998 at the age of 45; housewife and mother

"Looking back over my experience, I realise how much I have gained. Having breast cancer was an opportunity to live my life to the fullest. This is not to say that I was dancing with joy when I heard the diagnosis. But you can learn that you are stronger than you thought. You just face it and let it flow over you. It does not define who you are. It is something that comes along, just like anything else, and you decide how to live through it. We don't get to choose when we are born or when we die, but we can choose to be happy and fully present in the time between the two."

Adelaide D. Key; diagnosed in 1978 at the age of 42; community volunteer, philanthropist

"I learned that I am my own best friend, and that the inner me is stronger and braver than I'd ever thought possible. I learned to feel comfortable saying 'yes' when someone offered to run an errand for me or to cook dinner. I learned to have naps in the middle of the day – first by setting the kitchen timer for ten minutes and making myself close my eyes until it buzzed. I learned that my two dearest friends know what to say and when to say it. I learned how important it could be to receive a telephone call or greetings card. I learned that it's really okay to cry, even in public. I learned how to leave a little present for myself on the seat of the car so it would be waiting for me after each chemotherapy session. I learned how to leave my spirit outside the door of the treatment room so that the chemo would hurt only the ghost I took in with me. Now I'm the one devoting herself to charity fundraising. Now I'm the one sharing my belief that a person who *used* to have cancer was wheeled out of the operating room and that the person in the recovery room is already a survivor. Now I'm the one offering to lend an ear and give encouragement."

Kathi Ward; diagnosed in 1994 at the age of 47; promotions executive

"How can cancer make life better? The answers are still coming, four years after my diagnosis. You learn to see that each person who enters your life is a potential gift, and that you are buoyed up by a web of beautiful souls. You learn to discard old acquaintances and unsupportive friendships, to weed out those relationships that 'don't work'. You learn to make space in a busy workday for moments of appreciation beauty and love. You learn to make choices that feed rather than drain you. You learn to take care of yourself, to take naps, eat good food, drink water, go to bed early. You learn to pamper yourself – to read only books you like, take walks, go out into the countryside more often, have massages and healing treatments. You take time for art, for tea with friends, for crafts, reading or whatever it is that nurtures you and heals."

Deborah Pierce; diagnosed in 1997 at the age of 48; architect

"I'm tremendously grateful for all I learned from breast cancer. Yet the journey for me is not best expressed by the term 'survivor'. I'd rather call myself a 'breast cancer emerger', because I emerged from it a different person. I didn't just survive. I became someone new, someone better. I became a person who believes in the power of hope and who understands the importance of opening her heart and inviting love to come in."

Holly Marion; diagnosed in 1996 at the age of 49; fundraiser

Acknowledgements

....

I can write entire books without blinking, but putting together an acknowledgements page when there are so many people to recognise – now *that* is daunting. But I've run out of time. My publisher needs this part *yesterday*. So, here goes.

Since its inception, *UPLIFT* has been a grass-roots project. It is therefore fitting that my acknowledgments start and end with everyday people. Some of those – like Bobbi Kolton, Sue Rabin and Cindy Teeple – went above and beyond the call of duty in drawing attention to this project. I don't even know the names of some of the others who spread the word, but I do know that the following people played a part and deserve my thanks: Carol Baggaley, Jane Bender, Dale Berthiaume, Karen Boml, Martin Bradley, Marilyn Brier, Louise Broach, Jeanne Bryner, Robin Homonoff, Autumn Hughes, Treazure Johnson, Cristy Peck, Lucy Pino, Martha Raddatz, Jane Salk, Linda Saulnier, Suzanne Schmidt, Ellen Beth Simon, Jensie Shipley, Lynn Smith, Phyllis Stoller, Claire White, Cindy Wilkins, Susan Wornick and Nancy Zlotek.

My thanks to the wonderful women and men who disseminated information about *UPLIFT* through their medical facilities and support networks: Peggie Barten at Good Samaritan Diagnostic Center North in Florida, Deb Belfato at Susan G. Komen Center in New Jersey, Corinne Cook at Inova Alexandria Hospital Cancer Center in Virginia, Wanda Diak at Cancer Hope Network in New Jersey, Kathy Dorner at the Cancer Center at Arlington Hospital in Virginia, Julie Durmis at Dana-Farber Cancer Institute in Massachusetts,

James Dye at Christ Hospital Cancer Center in Ohio, Leslie Dykhouse at Fairfax Radiology Center in Virginia, Joan Frier of SHARE in New York, Francine Halberg at Marin Cancer Institute in California, Marsha Komandt at Inova Fairfax Hospital in Virginia, Catherine Owens at Carol G. Simon Cancer Center in New Jersey, Susan Sharp at Julius Hermes Breast Cancer Center in Virginia and Helen Maurice at UConn Cancer Center in Connecticut.

Massachusetts General Hospital has been part of my life since my mother was treated there when I was a child. Though I always knew that it would remain part of my life medically, I never dreamed that there would be a professional crossover, yet that has happened with UPLIFT. So, my huge thanks to all at Mass General who helped spread word of this project, beginning but not ending with those in the Development Office: Amy Fontanella, Beth Alterman and Peggy Slassman. A very special, very personal thanks to Dr Barbara L. Smith, who not only saved my life surgically, but saved me professionally by reading UPLIFT in manuscript form and catching several near-howlers.

I am particularly proud of – and grateful to – the writing community. Granted, writing is a field in which women are prominently represented, and women feel breast cancer most directly. Still, the eagerness of members of this community to help with UPLIFT touched me deeply. I thank Elaine Raco Chase, Sandra Brown and Dorothea Benton Frank. I thank Lauren Nichols, Jane Vaughan and Marcia Talley. I thank Blanche Marriott and the New England Chapter of the Romance Writers of America. I thank the readers of my novels – women like Nikki Provenzano, Lytrice Mains, Susan Edmondson and Diane Williamson. Five thousand of my most loyal readers were among the first to learn about UPLIFT and though many of them have had no personal experience with breast cancer, they sent information on this project to anyone and everyone they knew who has.

And then there's the publishing world in New York. UPLIFT would not be the book it is today without the enthusiasm, support and expertise of Judith Curr and Karen Mender of Pocket Books. My editor, Tracy Bernstein, always concise and smart and quick to respond, was a joy to work with. Michael Korda, of Simon and Schuster, gave me emotional support; Jodi Reamer, of Writers House, gave me technical support. My thanks to all of these wonderful people.

I am deeply indebted – always, but more so with this book for reasons that she knows – to my agent, Amy Berkower. If *UPLIFT* could not have happened without my attaining the success with my fiction that I have, Amy has to take some of the credit. She is a skilled advocate who has shepherded my career warmly and wisely.

Legally, I thank William Eisen, who gave generously of his time and expertise for this project. Fauzia Burke did an incredible job of publicising *UPLIFT* over the World Wide Web; more traditionally, Barry Michaelson supervised the printing of the material needed for a project like this and Diane Charron saw that everything was posted. Scott Mason saved me countless hours and many headaches by typing much of *UPLIFT* on to disk.

Claire Marino has been my webmaster since I first ventured into the realm of websites in 1998 with *www.barbaradelinsky.com*. Just as she designed and maintains that site, so she is the ongoing force behind *www.teamuplift.com*. Without this site – without Claire herself – *UPLIFT* would not be what it is.

Wendy Page is my assistant extraordinaire. Always a lifesaver with regard to my usual work, she has gone beyond the call of duty with regard to *UPLIFT*, which involved keeping track of so many names and submissions and sources that I would have long since sunk in the mire had she not been fully in charge at her end. For this and much more, I thank her from the bottom of my heart.

How to mention "heart" without mentioning my family? Husband, sons, daughters-in-law – each has contributed to *UPLIFT* in his or her own special way. In case you haven't guessed it, my family is my life. The infinite patience, unremitting enthusiasm and steady love of these people have seen me through far more than breast cancer and *UPLIFT*.

So now, have I failed to mention others? No doubt about it, if only because *UPLIFT* was such a word-of-mouth project that friends told friends, who told other friends. I doff my hat to you all.

Last, most of all, I acknowledge the women and men of *UPLIFT* – survivors all – who put their hearts and souls into writing to me and whose words constitute the body of this book. I am in awe of their courage and generosity. If goodness counts for anything, they will live long and well!

An Invitation from *UPLIFT*

Please join us! Once you've read *UPLIFT*, you'll have thoughts of your own about what helps and what doesn't. Make a note of these thoughts on the pages that follow. As many of the original *UPLIFT* submitters have pointed out, this can be therapeutic. Taking it a step further, if you would like to share your ideas, you can make an entry in the guest book at the *UPLIFT* website, *www.teamuplift.com*, or send them to me c/o *UPLIFT*, PO Box 812894, Wellesley, MA 02482-0026, USA.

For your convenience, I have included the general guidelines that were followed by the original contributors to *UPLIFT*. Keep in mind, though, that these are only suggestions. You may have already discovered dozens of other topics that relate to having breast cancer. The following guidelines are simply to get you thinking. My only request is that you be . . . well, uplifting!

I have what!?
   What was the most constructive thing you did after hearing your diagnosis?
   What was the most helpful thing someone else did for you upon learning of your diagnosis?

Whom did you tell, when and why?
   Did you tell your children?
   Did you tell your boss?

How did you tell the person you most feared telling? What made it easier?

Sister, friends and bosses . . .

What single most practical thing did a friend or family member do to help?

What single most helpful thing was done for you in the workplace?

How did you juggle cancer and work? What little tricks helped?

What about the men in your life?

How did they react to your bout with breast cancer? (Can I have a quote from them too?)

Husbands? Lovers? Sons? Brothers? Friends?

Hair today?

What most raised your spirits when your hair began to fall out?

Did you wear a hat when you had no hair? If so, what kind worked best?

Tell me about being bald. Tell me about wigs. Tell me about growing new hair.

When the going gets tough, do the tough go shopping?

What was your favourite piece of clothing during treatment, and why?

What single purchase most lifted your spirits?

How did you overcome the self-consciousness of undressing in front of others?

What was . . . what did . . . what is . . . ?

What kind of food helped curb nausea during chemo? Gave you energy? Gave you a lift?

What did you do with the tattoos on your body when radiotherapy was over?

What made you feel the most feminine during this time? The most sexy?

What did you do to show people that you were still alive and well?

What helped pass quiet times in lieu of worrying? A hobby, perhaps? If so, what and why?

What one person, place or thing made you feel most in control?

What was the funniest thing that happened to you during all this?

What is the single most important piece of advice you would give to a friend going through what you did?

A walk in the park . . .
What physical challenges did you face during rehabilitation? What helped most? Who helped most?

What sports did you do before breast cancer? After? How did it help?

In what ways is your post-cancer body better than your pre-cancer body?

Please do not . . .
Recount your diagnosis or treatment.

Offer medical advice.

Discuss your doctor, hospital or health plan.

Dwell on the negative.

Again, do not be limited by the above. If you have been personally touched by breast cancer, you no doubt have many more ideas than those listed here. Think about your experience or that of the person whose experience you've shared. What practical advice would you give to a friend who is going through this now? What nuts-and-bolts kind of hints can you give? What words of encouragement of an upbeat and useful nature? Can you tell me how having had breast cancer has improved your life?

Breast Cancer Organisations

UK

Against Breast Cancer
B363 Curie Avenue
Harwell International Business Centre
Oxon
OX11 0RA
Tel: 01235 820777
Email: info@aabc.org.uk

ABC aims to increase survival after breast cancer through new research into cancer vaccines and advice on diet and lifestyle changes.

Breakthrough Breast Cancer
Kingsway House
Kingsway
London
WC2B 6QX
Tel: 020 7405 5111
Fax: 020 7831 3873
Email: info@breakthrough.org.uk
www.breakthrough.org.uk

Fund raises for research into causes, prevention and new treatments. Currently establishing the first UK centre wholly dedicated to breast cancer research, in partnership with the Institute of Cancer Research.

Breast Cancer Care
210 New Kings Road
London SW6 4NZ
Tel: 020 7384 2984
Email: info@breastcancercare.org.uk
www.breastcancercare.org.uk

National organisation offering free information, help and support. Services include: free helpline, information, volunteer services and prosthesis fitting service.

Cancer BACUP
www.cancerbacup.org.uk

One of the most comprehensive cancer sites on the Internet — provides information, counselling and support to people with cancer, their families and friends through specialist cancer nurses.

The Lavender Trust
Kiln House
210 New Kings Road
London
SW6 4NZ
Tel: 020 7384 4617
Fax: 020 7384 4610
Email: ltf@breastcancercare.org.uk

Support for younger women affected by breast cancer. Based at Breast Cancer Care.

Tenovus
43 The Parade
Cardiff
CF24 3AB
Tel: 02920 482000
Fax: 02920 484199
www.tenovus.com

Provides information on cancer and emotional support for patients and their families.

UK Breast Cancer Coalition
Suite 1D
Broadway House
112 – 134 The Broadway
Wimbledon
SW19 1RL
Tel: 020 8543 4455
Fax: 020 8543 5577
Email: info@ukbcc.org.uk
www.ukbcc.org.uk

The UK Breast Cancer Coalition is the leading organisation dedicated to improving breast cancer services through patient advocacy.

Australia

iSource National Breast Cancer Centre
Locked Bag 16 Camperdown NSW 1450
Australia
Tel: 02 9036 3030
Fax: 02 9036 3077
International: +61 2 9036 3030
Email: directorate@nbcc.org.au
www.nbcc.org.au

Provides information, contacts and support for those affected by breast cancer.

South Africa

Cancer Association of Southern Africa
CANSA
National Office
PO Box 2121
Bedfordview
2008
Tel: (011) 616-7662
Fax: (011) 622-3424
www.cansa.org.za

Provides information and advice on all forms of cancer.